As the title of this book implies, it is a love story, but one in which a cruel disease becomes the enemy. It could have been any terminal illness. However, I would have been missing an opportunity if I had not used it to inform the reader about the unique cruelty of motor neurone disease (MND). In whatever context you decide to read this book, whether it is to learn more about MND, or just for the story, or because you too have lost someone you love in tragic circumstances, I hope you will, at the very least, find it thought provoking. It is harrowing in places, because I have told it as it was. I have let you into our life – the pain and the joy.

True Love
Cruel Fate

Nicola Wood

A Tribute to my Partner who died of Motor Neurone Disease

Seven Arches
Publishing

Published in July 2009
By Seven Arches Publishing
27, Church Street, Nassington, Peterborough PE8 61QG
www.sevenarchespublishing.co.uk

A catalogue record for this book is available from the British Library

Graphics by Alan McGlynn

Printed in Great Britain by imprintdigital.net

ISBN 978-0-9556169-7-6

Acknowledgements

I need to thank Alan for his irritating hoarding habit. Without this I would not have been able to piece together so much of his life. He would hoard anything from odd bits of wood to bills, papers and clothes. After so many years of living with this, the habit rubbed off on me. In writing this book I have sensed him saying, on many occasions: 'I told you; you should never throw anything away – you never know when it might prove useful!'

I would also like to thank all those friends and relatives who helped me to write this book by filling in some of the gaps that I needed to fill, and those who helped me to bring it to its final stage for publishing.

I will always be grateful to everyone who supported, or tried to support us, during Alan's illness, and to those who continued to support me after he died.

Contents

Foreword

At times, Nicola Wood's words are emotionally painful but they never deviate from the reality of living with motor neurone disease. Throughout True Love Cruel Fate we are conscious of the shadow that MND can cast over lives.

As Nicola shows, following the frightening diagnosis of MND trying to find out what services and support is available, under what rules, and to co-ordinate this around an individual's needs can be an immense burden for everyone affected by the disease. Her frank and moving account covers the whole spectrum of the complex issues that the progression of MND can bring. Those who have been affected by the cruelty of MND will no doubt be able to identify with aspects of Nicola and Alan's experiences. But this is not just a book for those who have first hand knowledge of sharing their life with this disease.

Health and social care professionals will gain an honest and at times uncomfortable insight into the real need for effective support and care. The need for families to be in contact with a single person – a 'key worker' within a multi-disciplinary team – who can ensure that all the support and care, no matter who provides it, is properly planned and coordinated.

We must never forget that everyone's experience of MND is unique and so too are their needs. True Love Cruel Fate encapsulates the MND Association's belief that for people living with MND it is essential that they understand what options for care, treatment and day-to-day living are open to them and that importantly their voices are heard. The Association helps them to do this whilst also providing equipment and funding to improve their quality of life.

Jane Skelton, MND Connect, MND Association

Preface

I wish it had not been necessary to write this book. It would have meant that Alan had not had motor neurone disease and that he would still be here with me now.

When he died, my first feeling was one of relief. At last the suffering was over, and he was at peace. I felt calm. It was as though I was floating, and nothing around me was real; I had switched to automatic pilot – becoming numb. Of course, I was in shock, and that was how I would stay for the first two to three months afterwards. Having lost, in the cruellest way, the person who was both the centre of my world and the only world I wanted, shock provided a natural protective cloak. But it could not last forever. I knew I had to start coping with reality, and it was then that the protective cloak left me; for a while I thought I would go stark, staring mad. At times, I think I was.

Others had lost too: a friend, a father, a grandfather and a brother. But they had not lost the person who had been the centre of their world. And they had not had to watch him dying in slow motion, as I had done – every cruel humiliating stage of the disease. The means to come to terms with my loss was going to have to come from within. I could not expect others to understand.

But first I would have to face the disease again. It hit me, out of the blue, with that picture of Alan, in the latter stages of MND. It had been lurking in the recesses of my mind, waiting to jump out at me. Now it wouldn't go away. That was what made me scream again. I had become very good at screaming while Alan was ill, but this was the first time since he died. I screamed and screamed. The pain was so great that I had to scream. All the memories of his illness came flooding back. They wouldn't go. I went on screaming until I was too tired to feel the pain. That was when I sat down, on the bottom stair, with my face in my hands and wept. Grief had kicked in. With it came all the anger I had felt, while I waited for the disease to finish consuming Alan.

I had lost 'my other half' to a disease which, over nearly two and half years, took his life piece by piece, in front of my eyes. The grief was overwhelming. What a small word for such a multitude of emotions. We had been through living hell together, but we had not survived together. The disease was gone, but I had returned from the battlefield alone. Everything I had been fighting for was lost. I had survived, but the disease had taken Alan. Nothing could ever have prepared me for the way I felt. Our world had disappeared in all but memories, and I was finding even those difficult to locate amongst the mental debris left by the disease.

There were long periods of the day when I would move through the house, hunting through drawers, through the loft, anywhere that I might find a little piece of Alan. I was looking for anything that would bring him back, and for the memories of life before the illness. I hoped for something tangible. The thought that he would never walk through the door again was incomprehensible.

I tried counselling. It helped, and I was lucky it was available. I was offered anti-depressants. I refused. Maybe they would have helped, but that wasn't my way. Instead I chose to write. Initially, it was just my thoughts. It was the only way I could begin to stop them endlessly going round and round in my head. At that point, I was trying to write down everything that had happened in that last part of Alan's life, trying to write it out of my system. But at the same time, I needed to find the person Alan was before he was diagnosed with MND – my Alan, not what the disease had made him.

That was how this book started. I felt compelled to tell our story. In the process of writing, it occurred to me that, if other people read our story, something good might come from the dreadfulness of it all. I hope our story will give you some idea of what it was like to live with MND. You can never know exactly what it was like. For that, you would need to go through it yourself. Hopefully, this book will be the closest you will ever get. But if you are, or ever do find yourself, in a similar situation, I hope this book will be of help, and offer you some comfort that you are not alone in what you feel.

People said: 'You were wonderful. How can you feel guilty?' Well, as you read this book, you will see. And, of course, although we went through the disease together, only I survived. It took a long time to begin to come to terms with this. It remains work in progress.

Although the thoughts expressed in this book are my own, I have little doubt that they echo Alan's in many ways.

This book became a means for me to start repairing the damage inflicted on me by the disease. With each happy memory, pulled from the depths, I managed to patch together another piece of my heart. Of course, I will never be the same person. A key part of me will always be missing. However, writing this book has shown me that Alan left me with so much of his life, before the disease, to treasure and keep with me for the rest of mine.

It is a real life story of love and happiness. It is a story about the fear of pain and loss, and also the effect on two people of a cruel terminal disease. It is the story of a very human relationship.

I was Alan's partner for the last twenty-six years of his life. It was over half of mine, and more than a third of his life. By telling our story, I hope to pay tribute to the man I loved so much – a kind, gentle, wise and thoughtful man with an infectious love of life. Our lives might have been very different, if we had not met. I am glad we did, and somehow even our meeting seemed like fate.

First Symptoms and Diagnosis

Alan was standing in his dressing gown, his back to the washing machine; we were talking together in the kitchen, as we so often did. I don't know if it has something to do with the warmth of this part of the house, but it always seems to act like a magnet. It was the room where we had most of our meals, and talked about things going on in our lives. He was joking, making us both laugh, and looking at me with those unforgettable smiling, twinkling eyes. It made me so happy seeing him like this - healthy.

I started to go towards him. How I yearned for him to say 'I love you' and for one of his everything-will-be-alright hugs. It had been such a long time since he had been able to give me a hug. I could see he wanted this too but, just as he started to lift his arms towards me, he disappeared.

I woke up with a start. It was a dream; he wasn't there after all; he couldn't be; he was dead.

25 November 2003

I took Alan to the station, on my way to work. It was a Tuesday morning.

He was a stickler for timekeeping. If he said we needed to leave at 9.00 am, that meant being in the car and driving, not putting your shoes on to leave the house. Before I got to know him better, he would be standing at the door, calling: 'Come along Nicola.' I had always been quite a good timekeeper, and I couldn't understand what all the fuss was about. As far as I was concerned, we still had five minutes to go. Once I knew what he meant, I was ready and in the car at the appointed time. This avoided any rise in blood pressure (his not mine), something that, I always felt, contributed to his heart problem.

He suffered from atrial flutter and fibrillation* which first came to light when he was carrying my skis for me, on a skiing holiday in Kitzbühel. He would pull my leg and say it was carrying my skis which started it. More than likely he was born with it, but it only became apparent in Kitzbühel. Once we knew it wasn't life-threatening, it was less of a worry. However, the attacks became more frequent and increasingly debilitating, as he got older. It used to leave him feeling very tired.

After dropping him off, I had a twenty-minute drive. Normally, I would have been looking forward to the day, and thinking about what I might be asked to do. Every Tuesday, if we weren't away somewhere, I worked as a volunteer for a gardening charity. I had done this since I stopped paid employment, in 1998. It gave me an interest of my own, but didn't get in the way of my being with Alan, after he retired.

I could be asked to do any one of a number of jobs at the garden. As it was a beautiful sunny day, if a little on the cold side, I would probably be asked to help map one of the flower beds with a colleague. The gardens occupy a large area, so making lists of all the plants, and where they are in the individual beds in the garden, enables us to keep stock of everything, more or less. This is useful for visitors to the garden, who might want to see an example of something they would like to grow at home. It is a task I enjoy still, not just because it is outside, but also because I can learn the names of plants, and see how they work in the overall design of a flower bed; the mix of evergreen and deciduous trees and shrubs, interspersed with flowering perennials, coming together so easily that it is hard to imagine the effort that has gone into creating the scene.

But this morning was different. All I could think about was what Alan had told me the evening before. We had always been so lucky, but now this bombshell. He had been to see a neurologist at the hospital. He had gone on his own, because we thought the appointment was just for a routine referral to have an MRI scan.

'Do you want the good news first, or the bad news?' he had asked, when he came home. He had even managed a chuckle. I suppose he was trying to make light of it, trying to be strong. As I drove the car through the winding country lanes, I was still trying to think what the good news was.

The neurologist had told him that he thought Alan had motor neurone disease (MND)* He had spotted the fasciculations in the muscles around Alan's shoulders. Under the skin, the muscles were rippling. They looked a bit like the surface of a pond when a pebble is thrown into the water. But unlike the ripples on the water, these wouldn't stop.

Both Alan and I knew exactly what this meant: it was a death sentence, and a frightening one at that. In 2002, we had followed the case of Diane Pretty who had died that year of the very same disease. She had fought through the courts, with her husband, for the right to be able to choose medical help to die. She wanted to be able to die at the point when she considered she no longer had any quality of life. We were particularly moved by her situation, and both felt that we would want the same. In fact, we had said to each other that, should either of us ever be in a similar situation, we would want help to die, at the moment of our choosing.

I simply couldn't believe that, less than two years on, Alan actually had this horrible disease – a hopeless, cruel terminal illness. I was shocked to the core. I tried to tell myself that the neurologist could have got it wrong. He was referring Alan for tests, so surely he must have some doubts about his diagnosis? I kept thinking, how on earth did he drive home on his own? When he told me the news, I had said, 'whatever happens we are in this together' – whatever that meant; after all, he was the one with the disease; but I would learn with time. He was trying to be strong, but I could see the vulnerability and fear in his eyes. Somehow, but I didn't know how, I would have to be strong with him. Neither of us had slept much the night before. I had managed not to cry, not until I left Alan at the station. But nothing would stop the flow of the tears, now that I was on my own in the car. I cried all the way to work. I was about to lose the most important person in my life, in a dreadful way. The pain in my heart was so great I thought it would break into lots of tiny pieces.

I parked in the car park at work: I don't know how I got there. I looked into the rear view mirror at my eyes, red and swollen; I had to do something about them before I went into the office. I didn't want to tell anyone about the diagnosis – not yet. It could still be wrong.

I went to the cloakroom in the car park, and put cold water on my eyes. I looked at them again in the mirror. Not too bad. I took a few deep breaths, stepped outside and walked through into the gardens – there was still plenty of time before I was due to start work. As I walked, I tried to think about something else, noticing that the leaves had now gone from the trees. High hedges – also bare of leaves – sheltered the garden from the harsh weather, and divided it into smaller areas. Each area distinct from the other – the bright colours of the rhododendrons and azaleas at the end of spring; the contrasting and complementary colours of the mixed borders in summer; the wild garden with its plentiful trees and leaves turning to rich autumn colours of copper, yellow and orange after the first frosts: all were part of a grand design.

Design had brought us together and it became a part of our lives. Alan noticed fine detail. He had an eye for beauty in all its forms. He saw it in the design of a motor car, in a building, or in a landscape. When he saw such things as the dew glistening on a spider's web in the early morning sunlight, he would run upstairs to fetch the camera, so he could capture it before it disappeared.

We had first met in 1979, a year or so after I gained my degree in Business Studies. Getting a degree was not forecast for me during my early education. The head of my first school had told my parents I would never be degree material. I was late learning to read. Nevertheless, they always expected me to try hard, and failure never went down well. So I graduated, apparently against the odds, and I don't remember my parents telling me they were proud. I am sure they were pleased, but possibly they simply expected it of me, because of all the money expended on my education. The lack of parental encouragement, especially from my father, undermined my confidence all through my life until I met Alan. He gave me everything that was lacking in my relationship with my father. I don't blame my father, because I don't think fatherhood came naturally to him. He didn't really know how to nurture confidence in a child. He had a lot of good qualities, but he had not shaken off the damaging effect of his own father. My grandfather was a bully who took the Victorian view that girls were not worth educating.

My father once told me, that if I didn't pass my eleven-plus exam, and get a place at one of the high schools, I would be a failure. I did fail. Well, I was a borderline pass, but as there weren't enough places at the high schools, I didn't get in; so it seemed to amount to the same thing, and it would have a profound effect on me in my future life. Although profound, the effect was not altogether negative. Hard work, determination, and a stubborn desire to prove I wasn't a failure, earned me the degree and everything else since.

After graduating, I landed a job as a marketing assistant with a local company, and lived at home with my parents in Plymouth. The company made pocket money toys – low priced play-kits for children – and my unforgettable contribution to the range was basket-weaving. The instructions were a nightmare! It was at this company that I met Alan. Part of my responsibility was to brief the design for the packaging. His company would then design the packaging, and fine-tune all the copy, including any instructions. Apparently, the basket-weaving instructions caused some amusement amongst his copywriting team, and over the years Alan would often pull my leg about having suggested this product for the range.

The first time I saw him, I was with my boss, Graham. We had travelled from Plymouth to London by train, for a meeting with him. His company was called Parlour Wood, taking his name and the name of his partner, Ron Parlour. Alan and Ron had originally worked together for another commercial design company, The Design Group, but they had both become disillusioned. A year or so after Alan had left The Design Group to join another venture, he and Ron got together to start Parlour Wood. That was in 1971. Although they retired in 1994, the company continued and they both maintained a shareholding.

My boss and I arrived for the meeting with Alan, at around eleven o'clock. He walked into the reception area, and held out his hand to greet us. He was looking straight at me, as he shook hands with both of us and immediately, his eyes attracted me. They were brown, slightly mischievous and kind. He was tall, but not very tall, with broad shoulders and a moustache. I am not keen on moustaches, but his made him look a bit like Burt Reynolds. He was wearing a smart navy suit. Underneath the jacket was a crisp white shirt, with an expensive silk tie. Wow!

We broke off from our meeting for lunch at a restaurant called the Genevieve. It was small, so there weren't many tables. The people seated at them were nearly all men, smartly dressed businessmen. It looked very sophisticated with its white tablecloths, highly polished cutlery and sparkling glasses.

Alan checked whether we all liked prawns, before he ordered a large portion for us to share. When the waiter brought them to the table, he placed them in the space he had already cleared, in the middle. The prawns were resting on a bed of crushed ice, on a large raised glass dish. I had never had prawns like this before. It would be one of the many things Alan would introduce me to, like caviar and wild strawberries and going to places like Claridges and the Ritz Hotel. It would usually be work accompanying and supporting him when he entertained clients. However, these were all experiences I would probably not otherwise have had. Sitting there, that day, having lunch at the Genevieve, I had no idea what the future had in store.

After the prawns, I had pigeon. I chose this because I thought it would be a bit like chicken. When I tried to cut through the bird, it slid across the plate and sent a dollop of sauce flying across the table; it landed on Alan's shirt. I stared, transfixed as the rich brown gravy slid down his perfectly white shirt-front. That's it, I thought. Now I've made a complete fool of myself.

'I'm so sorry!' I stuttered.

'Don't worry – it's nothing. They're often a little tough to get off the bone. Would you like me to cut it up for you?' he said kindly. I accepted willingly.

As I would later find out, Alan was twenty-two years older than me. He didn't look it, but I don't doubt that he represented something of a father figure. Over the years he would give me the feeling of security that I had missed so much in my childhood. Before I met him, fear of failure had been a significant driving force. He would become the driving force after that – always there, always supporting me.

Strange, how life works out. What if I hadn't taken that job? What if Alan and his business partner Ron hadn't set up Parlour Wood? Would we ever have met?

I was so wrapped up in my thoughts that I hadn't noticed the chill in the air. Suddenly, I felt it. It reminded me of the chill in my heart, and brought me back to the present.

I thought again of the vulnerability I had seen in Alan's eyes, the night before – fear and vulnerability. This was not like him. He was always in control of his life, and that was what made me feel safe. He wouldn't let anything harm me. I had caught a glimpse of the future in his eyes, and I didn't like it.

I started to wonder how he was getting on, alone with his thoughts. He was travelling up to London, to attend the Annual General Meeting of Parlour Wood. Still one of the shareholders, he liked to know what was going on – inquisitive as always – and it was an opportunity to meet up with Ron.

I imagined him sitting on the train, staring down at his hands. It was his hands that had started it all off, almost two months earlier, while he was playing golf.

His game had been going reasonably well, until he needed a pee. Fortunately, it was a friendly match. I can't remember exactly who he was playing with that day, except that a friendly game usually included Roger and Rodney, and the three of them formed part of the 'Rat Pack', as they had come to be known at the club. It was a description that always tickled Alan.

'I just need a pee,' he had mentioned to his chums, before he went off behind a tree. Then he found he couldn't undo the zip of his trousers. 'I couldn't feel the ends of my fingers! I think my hands got cold. I had to come out from behind the tree to get help, and wasn't sure I would make it back to the tree in time. Luckily I did,' he managed to say with a smile of amusement. The others apparently managed a good laugh at his expense, and I laughed along with Alan, as he related what happened.

Later, when Alan told the story to his osteopath, he suggested it would be a good idea to have an MRI scan, just to check there was nothing wrong with his neck. The doctor referred him to see a neurologist privately, so the scan could be done quickly. It was at this appointment that he was given the diagnosis. No warning, no gentle bedside manner, no nothing. Just 'I think you have motor neurone disease.'

The neurologist had gone on to say he would arrange for the MRI scan and an EMG* test but it was unlikely that he could be wrong. What Alan's response was, I don't know. He left the hospital, and I wondered how long he had sat in the car before driving home, trying to work out how he would tell me. How do you tell someone you love that you have a terminal illness – this terminal illness? He must have asked himself: 'Will Nicola be able to handle it? – not everyone can, and what will I do if she can't?'

I walked into the office. 'Good-morning. How is everyone?' I asked as usual, as though nothing in my life had changed.

26 November 2003

Concorde took off from Heathrow.

From the garden of our house, we watched her ascent. We often went outside to watch this beautiful jet plane flying overhead, drawn by the noise of her supersonic engines. But, there was something poignant about this particular time. We followed Concorde as she climbed higher and higher, like a paper dart in the sky. She was at the start of her journey to Filton Airfield, at Bristol. There she would touch down for the last time.

So much had happened since we had first moved into the house, nearly twenty years ago. Were we now set on the final part of our journey together?

As we watched the plane streak across the sky, I am sure we were both thinking of the times Alan had flown on Concorde to New York. He loved flying. He had served his National Service in the RAF (from 1952 to 1954). He was sent to Egypt, to the Canal Zone, serving his time as a duty clerk – and playing rugby for the British Forces team. He possibly hoped he would learn to fly, but the only time he flew during this period, was to and from Egypt. He started to learn to fly much later in life, getting his student pilot's licence, in 1972.

Flying still gave him a thrill, and he felt privileged to have flown on Concorde. He travelled on her a couple of times to New York. He went there once a year, for the annual Toy Fair. It always took place around Valentine's Day.

The last time he went to New York for the Toy Fair, I travelled with him, but not on Concorde, because of the added cost. It was 1990 and our first Valentine's Day together. In previous years he had gone off with my cards to him in his suitcase, leaving me to find his cards under his pillow.

Our flight got off to an exciting start! Soon after take-off, we were advised by the pilot that we were flying on one engine. It would be necessary to fly over the Irish Sea to dump most of our fuel, before returning to Heathrow. We finally took off for New York later that night. When we arrived in the early hours of the morning, our room in the hotel, The Algonquin, had been let. As luck would have it, however, one of the floors was free - scheduled to start being refurbished after the weekend. The hotel was able to let us have one of the suites on that floor.

We woke up in our very comfortable suite in the morning, feeling like zombies, but unlike Alan, I didn't have to go to work. I was free to explore the city that I had never been to before. I decided the quickest, and easiest way to do all the tourist sites, was via one of the city orientation tours. Even though I was on my own, I enjoyed this introduction to the sights and sounds of bustling New York. On the way, we went past a place called Sweet Basil's, in Greenwich Village. The guide on the coach told us that it was renowned for its 'jazz brunch' on a Sunday. Apparently Doc Cheatham, a legendary trumpeter, who accompanied blues singers such as Bessie Smith and recorded with Billie Holliday, played there. The club offered new talent an opportunity to be noticed, and Doc Cheatham would be providing their accompaniment that coming Sunday.

I made a mental note to suggest it to Alan. We had planned to spend Sunday in New York together, before flying back home on the Monday morning. We both liked jazz, and one of our first dates had been at Ronnie Scott's, the famous jazz club in London. I was sure it would appeal to him to go to Sweet Basil's. For the Sunday morning, I was going to book a helicopter flight over Manhattan Island. It was to be a treat for Alan for letting me go with him to New York. I thought Sweet Basil's would be the perfect follow on.

As it turned out, we didn't see much of Manhattan Island from the helicopter! We managed to squeeze in a bit of shopping at South Street Seaport, before taking a bus to Greenwich Village, and laughed for most of the bus ride about the fact that the seats we had reserved on the helicopter had been on the wrong side for the view. We had thought it would fly once round in one direction, then again in the other direction, so everyone would get a good view. We were mistaken, and spent the whole flight craning our necks in order to see over the passengers on the other side, and through their small window.

We stayed at Sweet Basil's until four o'clock in the afternoon. It was difficult for us to tear ourselves away even then. However, we were running out of time, and there were still things we wanted to see and do. We had decided to walk back to Central Park via the Rockefeller Centre, so we could watch the people ice skating, outside in the big open-air rink. By the time we got there, it was bitterly cold and late. We still couldn't go back to the hotel, though; not until we had taken a pony and trap ride. Our pony was called Jimmy and the driver was from Northern Ireland. We snuggled up under the blanket while we were driven round the streets of New York. A perfect end to a long and perfect day! We were both happy but exhausted. 'Time for the sandman, I think,' Alan said, as he bent down to kiss me, before putting his arm round me, for the short walk back to the hotel.

27 November 2003

I was making breakfast when Alan came into the kitchen. With words reminiscent of one of those US journeys into space, he said: 'I think we have a problem.' He had discovered fasciculations in the calf muscles at the back of his legs. I tried to put his mind at rest by telling him that we still didn't know for sure. We should wait for the test results. The rippling in his muscles could be a symptom of something else.

4 December 2003

We were advised that the first scan was fine, so no need to worry! But the consultant had asked for another scan, further down his back. What did all this mean? Alan had an appointment with his osteopath. The suspense was unbearable. He decided to take a copy of the initial scan along with him. The osteopath could see evidence of cervical spondylosis*. Could this account for the symptoms? It might. It would still be an unpleasant diagnosis, but not in the same league as MND.

8 December 2003

Alan had to go for the EMG test in the evening and the second MRI scan on Wednesday. We wouldn't get the full results until his next appointment with the neurologist.

18 December 2003

The day of the appointment with the neurologist arrived. This time we both went to the hospital. It was 6.45 in the evening when Alan was called in. I don't know why I didn't go in with him. Perhaps Alan wanted to go in alone, not knowing how he would react. But at least I was there. He wasn't alone like last time. I waited outside, praying harder than I have ever prayed for anything.

The consultant accompanied Alan back into the waiting area to tell me: 'It appears I was wrong.'

The results of the nerve conduction test suggested that everything was normal, while the MRI scan apparently indicated some evidence of cervical spondylosis. Just as the osteopath had said! You can't imagine the relief. But at the same time, I wanted to punch the neurologist on the nose for putting us through such agony. I controlled my anger, and decided to put it behind me. It wasn't important now. My prayers seemed to have been answered. The neurologist referred Alan to a neurosurgeon.

We went through Christmas full of hope. The death sentence had been lifted.

Christmas 2003

Christmases with Alan had always been a complete contrast to those of my childhood. When I was a child, my grandfather used to spend Christmas with us, and the atmosphere was never light or happy when he was around. Stern and authoritarian, he cast gloom over everything.

There had been that Christmas, when we were all sitting around the table, eating our turkey, when something made my sister and me laugh. We were probably being silly and pulling faces at one another. He told us off: 'Children should be seen and not heard. Besides, life is not a laughing matter.' Mum had been trying hard not to giggle as well, because she knew what he would say, and didn't want to encourage us. It left the three of us looking at each other uncomfortably; trying not to show how much we disliked this killjoy of an old man.

Alan's childhood Christmases, on the other hand, had been very happy and full of fun. They had treasure hunts for presents, and children were probably very much at the heart of things. For their first family Christmas when the Second World War ended, Alan's older brother, Lionel, organised for the two of them to provide some entertainment for the adults. He had to list what he wanted Alan to do via letter, because he was away at school in Solihull. He wanted them to put on a play and sing carols to celebrate 'the first Christmas of peace.'

Alan was a big kid when it came to Christmas. He would get up early on Christmas morning while I stayed snuggled up in bed. I liked to lie there enjoying the feeling of warmth, secure under the bedcovers, and listening to him - imagining what he was doing.

I would hear him putting on the kettle to make a cup of tea for us all – these days. my mother was always with us for Christmas. I would visualise him switching on the lights on the Christmas tree, and lighting the fire in the sitting room to make it feel festive and cosy. He always did this while he waited for the kettle to boil.

Alan loved lights on a tree at Christmas. I would decorate the one inside on my own, but we did the one in the garden together. We had it down to a fine art: I brought the lights down from the loft; Alan checked them before we took them outside; he stood on the ladder; I held on and fed him lengths of the lights to curl around the tree; every so often, I gave him a piece of wire to hold them in place. In the evening the lights were officially switched on! Christmas had started.

As I lay in bed on Christmas morning 2003, I heard the stairs creaking, letting me know that Alan was on his way up with the tea. He knocked on the door of my mother's room, opened it, and put her tea down on the bedside cupboard, as he wished her a 'Happy Christmas.' Then he came in with my tea. 'Happy Christmas, lovely.' All his cards to me, were tucked under his arm. I had placed mine to him in my bedside drawer the night before, and got them out while he was taking the tea into my mother's room. I had placed them on his pillow. He smiled as he saw them, and, after he put my tea down beside me, he got back into bed. We sat up in bed together, drinking our tea and opening our cards - just the ones to each other. We used to give each other lots of cards

15

with different messages inside; some funny, some plain silly, and the all-important ones that said 'I love you' – in different ways, with different words.

Later that morning, while we all got ready to go over to visit Alan's daughter Caroline, he kept the festive atmosphere alive by playing Christmas carols and songs. He particularly liked "Hark the Herald Angels" and Bing Crosby singing, "I'm dreaming of a white Christmas." Before we went, I set the timer for the turkey to cook.

This year we wanted to maintain the status quo more than ever. We didn't want anyone to know what we had been through, and we assumed that whatever Alan had wrong with him it was not MND. Alan's daughter lived ten to fifteen minutes away, with her partner, Reg and young son, James. We had been going over to her house on Christmas morning ever since the birth of James in 1992. There were always lots of presents to open, and mulled wine and 'nibbles' for lunch.

Eventually, we returned to our almost-cooked turkey; all that was needed was to cook the vegetables. But the highlight was always the Christmas pudding, which Alan turned into a great theatrical performance. I loved this.

He would turn out the lights in the dining room, and follow me into the kitchen to fetch the pudding. I turned it out onto a plate, and he doused it in brandy, while I returned to the table and Mum. We both waited there, in quiet anticipation, for Alan to bring in the pudding; the room lit only by the burning candles. As he carried it in, the brandy already lit and the flames dancing all over it, he sang "Good King Wenceslas." Mum and I joined in the singing, and we all watched the flames burning. This was a tradition of Alan's, possibly one that had been passed down the generations through his father. He loved this great act of theatre with the pudding every year, and this year it was worthy of an encore!

The day ended, as for so many families in the UK, with us all slumped in front of the fire and the television – Alan and I snuggled up to each other on one sofa, my mother laid out on the other. It was a normal Christmas.

31 December 2003

We celebrated New Year's Eve at the Golf Club, sharing a table with friends. The annual dinner dance is a light-hearted evening – exactly what we needed. Alan played in the club's Hogmanay Salver the next morning; business kept very much as usual. He managed to play quite well.

The old year could have ended worse. We could still be hopeful.

9 January 2004

We went to the bungalow in Cornwall for a week. I had never been able to feel the same way about the bungalow as Alan did. I should have loved it, because it was responsible for our first date. But it had been Alan's baby, not mine. Now, however, the feelings I held about the place were not as important to me. We would go there as much as Alan wanted. What if it turned out that he did have MND? If I had prevented him from enjoying something he loved, while he still could, I would never have been able to forgive myself.

Although we had been given a reprieve, the fasciculations and cold hands persisted. The initial diagnosis never really went away. I was trying to be positive. We both were – neither of us wanting the other to know our doubts. What if that first diagnosis turned out to be correct? We had learnt that MND could take a long time to be confirmed. Other possibilities have to be ruled out first.

From the A38 in Devon, we cut across Dartmoor to the A30. The latter taking us into Cornwall. I had spent many happy times on Dartmoor as a child – paddling in the cool shady rivers in the summer, and being carried on my father's shoulders, when I had become tired on long walks. My father was tall, and it was a special treat to see the views from this exalted position.

Now the moors reminded me of life. Sometimes the conditions can be harsh, sometimes you lose your way in the fog, but always there remains an underlying beauty that never goes away. I needed to hold on to this thought.

Alan started singing, "Remember Samantha – I'm a one girl guy". 'How about putting "High Society" on,' he suggested. I reached into the glove pocket for the disc. 'Good idea'. We both liked musicals; this one in particular. We sang along to Bing Crosby and Grace Kelly singing "True Love". My mind started to wander as the disc continued to play in the background.

It didn't seem that 23 years had gone by since that telephone call from Alan, asking me to go out with him for dinner. He was spending the weekend at his bungalow in Cornwall. It was mid-summer of 1980, while I was still working for the company in Plymouth. He came to pick me up from my parent's home – moustache shaved off, but still attractive; in fact more so. I was like a small child – very excited. My parents watched from an upstairs window, as we left in his car. I could see them looking out from behind the curtain, being nosy, and trying to get a glimpse of the man I had talked so much about, since that first meeting in London.

At his request, I had booked the restaurant. Not coming from the area, he didn't know the restaurants. I had chosen one in Modbury. It would mean another longish drive to the other side of Plymouth from where he had come, but the restaurant in Modbury had a good reputation. It was owned by one of the original TV chefs, whose name escapes me. The food was guaranteed to be good, and I wanted to impress Alan with my choice.

There were only a few tables and each one had a lighted candle on it. A log fire burned in the large granite fireplace, to the side of the room. It was cosy – romantic. It turned out that Alan was alone in Cornwall. He had just split up with his girlfriend. The evening went quickly. He was very easy company. We laughed a lot, and we seemed to have a lot in common, which surprised me, given the age difference. This turned out to be our first date, the start of a wonderful journey together.

From that first evening, we were like two magnets. Nothing pulled us apart – not until this disease.

We stayed at the bungalow for our first holiday together, in August 1981.

The extension, which Alan was having built on the side of the bungalow, was almost finished. It had been a painful and costly affair. I smiled to myself, thinking of his meetings with the builders. Perhaps this accounted for his dislike of building work. It may also have been the reason he delegated any building work we had done to our house, to me. He was good at delegating, as the people who worked for him would probably concur! Of course, he had to be a 'doer' as well, to have become so successful in business, but he was especially good at delegating.

With the building virtually complete, choosing furnishings was part of the holiday. When we were not doing this, we spent lazy days on the river, or went for walks.

Alan had a speedboat called "Dolphin" which he had bought from Ron. We used a rubber dinghy to get ourselves out to Dolphin's summer mooring, in the middle of the river. A short trip up the river would take us to a spot where we could stop the engine, and just bob up and down, letting the trees on the river bank shade us from the sun. Here we read a book or had a snooze. Other times we went out beyond the harbour to open up the throttle and have some fun. Once, Alan nearly lost me over the back when he did this. He forgot to warn me. I was sitting on the upright part of the seat. As the boat took off, I did too – luckily, only into the back of the boat, with my life jacket cushioning the fall.

We loved the walk from Golant to Fowey, which took us up behind the hotel, across the top of the hill; high above the railway line that carries china clay to the docks at Fowey. From the path, there is a beautiful view of the river, until it turns off to the right, to go down to Sawmills – a place which is used as a music-recording studio.

On one occasion, on this downward path, Alan tried to give me a piggy-back. He toppled under my weight, and we fell into a bed of stinging nettles, laughing.

The path climbs upward again through trees, across fields. Eventually it reaches the road into Fowey. Sometimes we kept on going, so we could get the ferry across to Bodinick, have lunch in the pub, get the ferry back again, and then the bus to the top of the road leading down to the bungalow. There was that other walk we liked to do, through the valley near Luxulyan, at bluebell time. The bluebell was probably Alan's favourite flower.

I had so many reasons to love the place in Cornwall. I tried so hard to love it. It did have a pretty garden, and I spent many happy hours working in it hoping the garden might help me to feel better about it. There was a rhododendron tree in the middle of the lawn, which we both loved. Every year it produced the most beautiful pale lemon flowers.

It was in a beautiful spot overlooking the River Fowey. But for all this, the bungalow lacked the same pull on me as it had on Alan. For me it was nothing to write home about, and despite redecorating, it always seemed oppressive inside. No matter how hard I tried to love the bungalow for Alan's sake, I couldn't.

Alan bought the property soon after he separated from his wife. It wasn't simply a place where he went to recharge the batteries. There was something more, something special. I can only guess that he may have used it to fill a hole in his heart. Leaving his wife meant that he could not have the relationship with his children he would have liked, and I think he used the bungalow to lessen the pain. It provided a distraction, and may have assumed greater importance as a result.

Quite late in our relationship, but back in the time when we were blissfully unaware that Alan would be diagnosed with MND, I had a rude awakening as to how important the bungalow in Cornwall was to Alan. We rarely argued, but on this occasion we did, and it was all because I wanted a new dining room table.

The one we had was more than twenty years old and needed repairing. The round top was supposed to be supported by the central pedestal, but over the years it had become wobbly, and if you leaned on one side the dishes slid towards you. I could have got it mended, but I had seen a table I liked in an antique shop. Unfortunately, it was necessary for me to ask Alan for the money, because I had given up paid employment a few years before.

Until the end of 1990, I had had my own successful career, responsible for the marketing, advertising and profitability of some well-known brands including the men's fragrance, Old Spice, and the indigestion remedy Rennie. The catalyst for giving up this career had been a particularly bad day. I had got back from the office, late as usual. Alan was putting his car away in the garage. He usually got home after me, but I was glad to find him already home. I pulled up on the drive, got out of the car and locked it. Alan could see something was wrong and asked, 'What is it?' That was the trigger for me to burst into tears. Choking them back, I answered: 'I can't do this anymore. I'm just not enjoying the job anymore.'

He put his arms around me, and said gently: 'You know you don't have to do it, not if you don't want to.' He was trying to tell me that he would take care of me; surely I knew that.

So I left my well-paid job as a marketing manager, but maintained my financial independence by working as an administrator for the local university. This job was much less stressful, and the hours not as long, so I could spend more time with Alan.

Then his desire to travel as much as possible during his retirement, made it difficult for me to continue to be employed. Naturally, I wanted to go with him, so I finally gave up paid work completely, in 1998. This meant that I was dependent financially on Alan for the first time in our relationship, and being fiercely independent, I didn't like having to ask for something, especially for a piece of furniture.

When I asked for the table, and he had said 'no' apparently it was because we couldn't afford it. I was upset and not a little aghast. His response had been a complete surprise. I knew he had been worrying about money, because the stock market was going through a bad time, but I couldn't see how things could be so bad that we couldn't afford a new table. He had always been generous, but then I had always been careful with money – a throwback to my childhood, when I had learnt to appreciate having, versus not having. I had not thought my request at all unreasonable. So I said, 'If things are that bad, perhaps we should sell Cornwall?'

He shouted back with real anger and emotion in his voice, 'you know how much I love Cornwall.' I did know he loved it, but the force of this reaction was completely unexpected, and out of character. It was the sort of reaction I would have expected if I had asked him to give up his children; an analogy closer to reality than I realised, otherwise I would not have chosen that moment to suggest selling the bungalow. I had never completely understood why he loved the place so much, and no matter how hard I tried, I never could have the same strength of feeling for it as he did. For me this was reserved for our home, back in Surrey. It was this home, the house that we had bought together in 1984, which was important to me. For me it was the only property I needed and I was wounded by his reaction.

The argument over the 'Bloody Dining Table', as the new table would become affectionately known when we finally bought it, was possibly one that needed to happen. We needed to clear the air and remind each other that two people formed this relationship.

But the argument over the dining table seemed irrelevant now, and since the argument and the ghastly diagnosis, I think the bungalow had started to become less important to Alan.

It all seemed so futile now.

21 January 2004

After only a few days back at home, we flew to Spain, to the Costa del Sol, to the apartment Alan bought in the same year we purchased our house.

It had been his decision to buy it. I had no strong feelings one way or the other, largely because it was intended to be a sort of investment. But it didn't turn out that way. Like Cornwall, it became another home, or to me, another burden. It was somewhere we had to spend time, to make it worthwhile having the property. It didn't represent the same financial burden as Cornwall, as it was not as old, and didn't require the same upkeep. For these reasons, I preferred it to Cornwall. I also preferred it because it was more of a holiday when we went there. It was built on a development. There was an administrator on site, to take care of anything that needed doing. Everything was familiar, so it was easy to slip into a relaxed frame of mind quickly, when we got there.

And whenever we went, I would remember the first time he took me to see the apartment, not long after he had bought it. He had a surprise in store for me, on the way. He told me to pack a separate overnight bag, and refused to tell me why. When we left the house, he didn't take the turning off the motorway to the airport. He kept driving towards London.

'Where are we going' I asked?

'It's a surprise! I can't tell you. You'll see when we get there.' He drove us to the front of the Savoy Hotel, and asked the doorman to park the car. We were staying the night at the Savoy and having dinner in the famous Savoy Grill!

Holidays would always be precious, but the ones we had shared in the early years were different. They had been an opportunity to relax on our own, in an otherwise hectic schedule. Later, when Alan retired, and I no longer worked, for a living, it was simply an opportunity to do things together. But Alan enjoyed being on the move all the time, whereas I didn't. We were different in this respect. Perhaps deep down he knew he didn't have as much time as he would have liked. 'Life is not a rehearsal,' he would say. I often wondered if he had a little bit of gypsy in his genes. Thus, holidaying at the apartment was a good compromise.

When I got off the plane at Malaga airport, I realised how much I needed this holiday; a two-week break completely away, a distraction from thinking about what the future might hold.

We did very little, apart from walking along the promenade beside the beach, at the nearby town of San Pedro, and eating out a lot. The weather was superb. The holiday helped us to feel more positive, greatly assisted by the fact that Alan's hands were better in the warmer climate.

12 February 2004

The appointment with the neurosurgeon came round. Alan had prepared a list of his symptoms to go through with him:

> *On waking, hands are warm – no problems – but within 10 minutes my hands go cold – although the rest of me is warm and the use of the thumbs becomes restricted, especially on the left hand.*
>
> *Left inside ankle always really hot and itchy.*
>
> *Wake up in the night with a burning sensation in the right foot.*
>
> *Left arm muscles beginning to show signs of wasting.*
>
> *Get very tired.*

The neurosurgeon deposited us firmly back in limbo. In his view, Alan did not have cervical spondylosis sufficiently badly to cause these symptoms.

He said he could understand why the first consultant had thought it might be MND, and suggested referring him back to that neurologist for more tests. But Alan told him, in no uncertain terms, that he wanted to be referred to a different neurologist. The first one's bedside manner had left a lot to be desired, and he wanted someone more sensitive.

23 February 2004

We saw the second neurologist. He was based at a different hospital from the one Alan had attended for that very first appointment. The hospital was also closer to our home, and smaller, which gave it a friendlier feel. This would all become important.

Alan was referred for blood tests and a brain scan. During the appointment, the consultant told us gently that there was a distinct possibility that Alan did have MND. By now it wasn't a surprise. He didn't hold out much hope that the tests would reveal any other cause for Alan's symptoms; they would eliminate other possibilities, and therefore, in all likelihood, bring us closer to confirmation of the original diagnosis.

We were just about to go off to St Moritz, and as usual we would spend my birthday there. Not the best start. The real emotional rollercoaster was about to begin and our lives would never be the same again.

26 February 2004

We took a morning flight from Heathrow to Zurich, and from there, the train to St Moritz.

How many years had we been winter holidaying in St Moritz? It must have been close to ten. The first time was so I could try cross-country skiing. I had lost my nerve for downhill skiing because of two accidents that happened before and during our first skiing holiday together. It was 1982, and Alan's son, Michael was with us on both occasions. Michael would have been about seventeen at the time. He had left school and was working in a warehouse. They skied together in a different class from mine.

The first accident happened when I was practising on a dry ski slope before our holiday. I lost my balance as I left the button lift and fell. I was knocked unconscious by the next button lift swinging into my head, as I tried to get up. The second accident occurred while I was standing on the nursery slope at the resort, minding my own business. Another skier lost control and ploughed into me. I spent the next three months on crutches, with a torn ligament in my knee. We had tried going to other resorts, with better snow, so I could attempt to get my nerve back, but I couldn't; so I thought the answer might be cross-country skiing.

St Moritz has good cross-country tracks. Alan was a good skier and loved to go skiing each year, which was why I had always hoped to conquer my nerves, but it simply wasn't happening for me, and whenever we skied together I felt as though I was holding him back. Hopefully, I would enjoy cross-country, and I could do this while Alan skied unimpaired. Unfortunately, I didn't enjoy it, or really get the hang of it. I found the 'glide' technique difficult and the whole thing hard work. While trying to control my cumbersome skis, I noticed some people were effortlessly walking in shoes. That's for me, I thought. I took to the many paths around the resort in some appropriate walking shoes. I never looked back. From then on, we returned to St Moritz every year. At last I had found a happy compromise.

The last part of the train journey to St Moritz is beautiful. Snow covered landscapes and trees. Frozen waterfalls emerging and hanging from the steep rock face of mountains; wide clear rivers running far below in the valleys. How many more times would we make this journey? I expect Alan was asking himself the same question.

When we arrived at the station in St Moritz, the hotel bus was waiting to meet us, as usual. Straightaway, we settled into the routine, which had become second nature to us, after so many years of going there. There were lots of familiar faces. Would we go back, would we see them again the following year?

Alan managed to ski most days and we walked on others – more or less as usual, except that Alan didn't ski for as long each day. His muscles became tired more quickly than in previous years. Perhaps it's his age. Let's hope, I thought.

I had two favourite walks. One took me down to the lake and through the pine woods, a beautiful winter wonderland, before crossing the railway line to the town of Celerina. This is where the Olympic Bobsleigh Run ends. I walked back to St Moritz, via the path that runs alongside the Cresta Run.

In 1994 I had persuaded myself to do the four-man bobsleigh with Alan. He was keen to do it, but his heart was playing up, so I didn't want him to go alone. I thought they wouldn't go too fast - not with tourists on board. How wrong could I be! I was behind the pilot with Alan behind me. He was in front of the brakeman. The driver's ribs must have been bruised at the end. I gripped him with my knees in terror, as we descended. I swear my helmet touched the ice when we virtually tipped on our side to take the bends.

Alan was typically cool. He tickled my neck on one occasion – a little way of saying 'I bet I know what you're thinking.' I was terrified! I think it was my heart that was fibrillating at the end. My knees shook so much that my legs could barely lift me up, out of the bobsleigh. I downed my reward – a glass of champagne – and took the certificate to remind me never to do anything so stupid again, even if Alan's heart was playing up!

This was not the first time, and nor would it be the last, that Alan forced me out of my comfort zone, and caused me to experience so much more in life as a result.

The other walk was my favourite. It enabled us to have lunch to-gether. So on one of the days I did this walk. I made my way up through the pure white, newly-fallen snow – feeling it crunch beneath each foot-step. It was important to savour this walk; just in case it was the last time. God, how much I hoped it wasn't. I stopped at the bench on the corner, where the path doubles back on itself, to look at the view. I was lucky that day, because there was no one else there. I sat down, thinking I would spend a moment enjoying the view, but instead found myself meditating on my life. Was this what fate had intended all along - that I should be looking after Alan at the end of his life. Somehow it seemed to have been equipping me to do this.

After all, at the age of fourteen or fifteen, I had had to look after my mother, when she was recovering from meningitis. At the time, her coordination and speech were severely affected, and she was unable to write. My mother remembered little about this time, as I realised on an occasion when I was talking to her about the 'three day week' and the power cuts which were going on when she was still recovering. She said she couldn't remember anything about blackouts or me studying for my A-levels by candlelight. She pulled through, largely due to her own stubborn determination (a trait I inherited) and some help from me.

I encouraged her to do the same dance classes that I did; the ones she had originally taken me to, in order to overcome my asthma – dance movements similar to modern ballet, are coordinated with breathing. My dance teacher – who taught well into her eighties – used to say, 'Don't forget to breathe;' we were all concentrating so hard on the dance steps that she couldn't hear any breathing. This always made us laugh, relax and breathe. The dance classes were called Margaret Morris Movement, after the person who developed it. The classes had helped me, and I thought they might help Mum; that the dance movements might help her coordination.

Slowly but surely she recovered; so much so that she took exams to teach others in Margaret Morris Movement, and with her nursing qualification, was able to give remedial classes for people with an illness or disability.

My mother's illness meant that, for quite a long time, I looked after the whole family; that is my mother, father and younger sister. I had to grow up rather quickly, at least in some respects. My school work suffered, and rather than be understanding, my father, strongly influenced by my grandfather's old-fashioned attitude towards women, suggested that I would have to leave my school. It was a private school and he didn't see the point of paying the school fees. It had been my mother who had fought for me to go to the school, and I had grown to love it.

The school was the only thing to give me any real sense of security. The teachers were great, and all my closest friends were there. It was a terrible threat, and so unfair as well; my father's insensitivity would have a profound effect on me.

Later, I looked after Sarah who had cerebral palsy. It was a school holiday job, through someone my mother knew, I think. I covered for a couple of weeks while her usual carer was taking annual leave. Unfortunately, her mother had multiple sclerosis, so she was unable to look after Sarah without considerable help. Fortunately they were a wealthy farming family, and able to employ people to help in their care, as well as affording all the latest equipment.

If it turned out that Alan did have this dreadful illness, as seemed likely, this would mean he would need me to help and look after him. Nursing was the last job I had ever wanted to do. The experience with my mother, and then looking after Sarah had simply served to confirm this. No, this was not part of my dream. He couldn't have this illness. What happened to the "happy ever after?" I started to cry, and had to take a deep breath to stop. I looked over at the beautiful view of the valley, and down at the town of St Moritz, nestled into the hill, immediately below where I was sitting. I tried to imagine the mountains around, enveloping me and giving me strength. It was time to get moving.

Continuing upwards, through the forest, I stopped to look at the snow hanging on the pine trees – stalactites glistening from the branches. I thought of the time Alan and I had travelled on the cable car up this very mountain. We had seen a stag deer pass beneath us. I always hoped to see one again when I was doing this walk. Would I see another today, just as magnificent, strong and standing his ground, with those huge majestic horns? Strong, just I hoped Alan would always be.

At the top, above the tree line, the path narrowed. I stopped again, and sat for a while on another bench. I still had time to soak up the view before I had to meet Alan, and I really didn't want the walk to end. If it went on for ever, Alan would always be there to meet me.

From this position, I could see further – the power of nature over man more apparent. Eventually, I got up and started off – the restaurant not far away. Coming to the point where the path opens up into a wide piste, I had to wait for a break in the line of skiers to cross in safety. Turning right after a little while, the path narrowed to lead through pine trees again. It could be icy and treacherous, but the new snow of the previous night meant the path was easy to walk along. After several climbs, the last one took me over the top to the restaurant. I just had to negotiate the well-worn wooden steps with the snow swept to one side to get to the restaurant terrace.

The hotel had reserved a space for us at one of the long wooden tables outside, because they are particularly popular with skiers, on a fine day like this one. The terrace was bathed in the warm rays of the sun. While I waited for Alan, I held my face towards it, trying not to think about anything. The empty moment was broken only by Alan's arrival. He had made it to the restaurant safely, and looked so healthy and happy. 'Hello lovely,' he said, smiling down at me.

We ordered a pizza to share. We could watch it being cooked, as the oven was on the terrace. While we waited we exchanged details of our morning, as usual. Looking at him, while we talked, I kept thinking surely he didn't have this terrible disease? It just couldn't be.

The next day he had a fall. Nothing serious, but he didn't have the power in his arms to get himself up. Some young skiers stopped to help him. He was lying in the bath, enjoying a nice hot soak, me sitting on the toilet seat, as he told me this. I knew what he was thinking. He was now having trouble doing up the buttons on his clothing, and he had had problems running across the road one day, to get to the entrance of the hotel. We were both thinking the same.

At the end of our holiday, we booked for the following year. We were trying to be optimistic; trying to block the enemy at the door. Even if Alan couldn't ski he could always come walking with me. We asked the hotel to make a note of our room on the booking, as usual.

18 March 2004

Bad news! It would be difficult to hide from the truth any longer.

Our appointment with the neurologist revealed there was nothing else which could explain the symptoms, only MND. We had been able to hope, until then, that there could be another explanation, but our hopes were rapidly dashed. Alan's brain scan was very good and the blood tests revealed no vitamin deficiencies.

The neurologist said he would refer Alan to a professor, a world authority on MND, at King's College Hospital, in London. This would give us a better idea of the prognosis.

25 March 2004

A bloody awful week in Cornwall!

So many emotions – anger, love, fear, insecurity, disappointment, and uncertainty were just a few of them! I didn't know what the near future would be like, let alone beyond, or how I was going to cope.

The only saving grace had been going to see my friend, Sara, while Alan played golf. Sara and I had been at school together. In fact, Sara probably saved my life when I was looking after the home while my mother was ill. I had been heating up some fat, ready to make chips, in the chip pan. I had managed to let it overheat and catch fire. I turned out the gas on the cooker, and threw water onto the pan. Yes, I threw water onto a burning pan of fat! Clearly I had not been paying attention in my science lesson. Sara walked into the kitchen, just in time to see what I was doing. She dragged me out as the pan blew up. I had a very lucky escape, thanks to her.

The last time I had seen her, we had met at Dartington Hall, which is in Devon – a forty-five minute journey from the golf course in Cornwall, where Alan played golf. Dartington is a place full of happy memories for me. I had played roly-poly on a long grass slope there, made daisy chains and climbed trees with friends as a very small child, even before I knew Sara. In my teens I still went there. I went with my first love, Shane, sometimes to listen to jazz or blues concerts, and sometimes just to walk around the gardens. I always grabbed any chance to go there, whenever Alan and I went to Cornwall, but not this time.

This time I just needed to be able to talk to Sara, without other people around. It was such a relief to talk to someone. I cried a lot.

On another day, when Alan was playing golf, I went to Truro. I usually enjoyed it, but it was so difficult watching people together, buying things for their homes, able to think about their future together. How long would we have?

A Time to Share and a Time to Tell

29 March 2004

Telling my friend Sara had made me realise that it would be helpful to tell my mother – whatever the prognosis. I wasn't finding it easy to share some of my feelings with Alan, which was an odd sensation.

My parents separated in 1984; the same year Alan and I bought our house. Parents and early experiences are the things that shape much of one's life – they make us what we are. My experiences, both early and more latterly, had left me closer to my mother.

My life began on an icy, cold night in February 1956, at a maternity home in Devonport, Plymouth. My father needed some persuasion to get my mother there, because I wasn't due for another two days, and he didn't understand that I was coming ahead of schedule. My mother couldn't make me wait! Reluctantly, he agreed to call for a taxi and together they went to the maternity home. On arrival, the taxi driver deemed it necessary to park away from the main door, because of the icy conditions. This left my mother and father risking the ice on foot. I believe he would happily have let her negotiate the ice alone, had she not pressured him by reminding him of her condition. At the door they were met by the sister, who had already been warned by telephone of their imminent arrival. As if on cue, there was an awful noise from inside. A mother, in labour, was making a very loud 'mooing' noise – like a cow. My father took fright and made a run for it, somehow avoiding falling over on the ice. My mother was left standing, looking blank, while the Sister tried to reassure her, by saying, 'Don't worry dear. We don't need him do we.' She said this more as a statement than a question. It appears the woman was 'mooing,' because she had been told it was better for her baby, better than screaming and shouting. My mother, having been left to cope without my father, adopted the more usual method – screaming and using colourful language.

So that was how I came into the world.

My earliest memory is of being pushed in my pram, along the pavement from our house in Beacon Park, Plymouth, by our neighbour. This neighbour looked after me when my mother needed to leave me, and I have happy memories of playing with her dressing-up box, sometimes with a small playmate, called Rosemary. Rosemary was the daughter of one of my mother's friends. We used to play together quite a bit. Sometimes she would come to stay overnight, and it was on one of these occasions that we had our potty fight. Rosemary thought she had the best potty, and I thought I did!

When alone with my mother, I used to like making a tent from a blanket over the dining room table. The food supplies, for my game of make-believe-explorer were the tins of food taken from the kitchen cupboards. The chairs, pushed under the table inside my tent, made suitable shelves. I would often play happily like this, while mum ironed.

I also remember putting my head through the balusters at the top of the stairs, until the day it got stuck. My mother decided that what went in must come out, and pulled while I screamed my head off – well out anyway. She was right. My head did come out, which saved calling the fire brigade, and messing up the balusters in order to cut me free.

My sister Fiona arrived on the scene four and a half years after me, and I can't say that I was overly enamoured by her arrival. I remember being taken into the 'front room', as it was called in those days. She was asleep in her carrycot, but started to cry when I looked at her. She was long and thin, and quite uninteresting. I decided – just as Alan's brother, Lionel had done, when meeting his baby brother for the first time – that she was clearly not something to play with, and left the room unimpressed.

Fiona suffered from severe asthma from a young age. I had it too, but not as severely as her. Instead I had eczema, particularly on my hands, with the consequence that some children at school didn't want to hold hands with me; they treated me as if I had leprosy, and this unkind treatment naturally upset me a great deal.

We moved to nearby Plympton soon after my sister was born – to a bigger house. Here we lived through the cold winter of 1962/63. The house was built on a steep slope, which meant the snow drifted down and piled up against the garage and front door, and we couldn't leave the house until it cleared, so no school or frozen school milk. Great!

My first memories of my father are at this house. I used to slide up and down his long legs, while he sat reading the newspaper in the living room, and I tickled his feet to get attention. He worked very hard, and didn't have a lot of time for his children, but when he worked from home he used to let me interrupt him, to record my voice into his dictating machine. We played this back together, and I remember we used to laugh at the way it sounded.

Sadly, my other strong recollection at this house, is of my parents arguing. In my family, there was quite a bit of unhappiness, and although there must have been some joy, we were never particularly good at sharing it. Sharing in the joy of family was something I only really encountered either with other families or with Alan.

Generally, I take after my mother, who is fairly practical. My father was not a practical man. He was more suited to a life of academia, not of a chartered accountant. The latter was what he did for a living, and it was the profession my grandfather chose for him. His head was either buried in books or up in the clouds. There was the time he decided we would all benefit from camping holidays together.

Much research was done to ensure he got it right – on paper. He bought the most up-to-date equipment; the most important piece being a trailer, which unfurled into a large tent. Reality, unfortunately did not match my father's plans. Driving along the main road, on our initiation trip, my mother smelt burning. We all, bar my father, seem to have been blessed with an acute sense of smell! My father stopped the car. The cause of the smell was traced by my mother, to smouldering wires, the ones that connected the brake lights of the car to those of the trailer. They had possibly started to smoulder when my father reversed. This would have been after we missed a turn, whilst we were trying to find the campsite. Fortunately, the campsite was not far away; so we un-hooked the trailer. My father and I pulled the trailer along the main road to the campsite. I wasn't very old at the time. This didn't stop him leav-ing me on my own to put up the tent. While I did this, with the help of some friendly people at the site, who had taken pity on me, he returned to my mother, younger sister and the car!

On another occasion, when my father displayed reluctance to use the self-service pump at the petrol station – the first time he encountered this new phenomenon – my mother decided she would fill up the tank. 'Oh, I'll do it,' she said, irritated by his reluctance to give it a try. She squeezed the trigger while reading the instructions. Following the in-structions to the letter, she hadn't yet put the nozzle into the opening for the tank! With Mum's hand firmly squeezing the trigger, a panicky voice suddenly shouted out over the loud speaker, 'Let go of the trigger!' Petrol was spilling out everywhere. I suppose the attendant was, under-standably anguished – all it needed was a match!

My father couldn't stop laughing, even when he had to pay. He was not a generous man, certainly as far as money was concerned, but on this occasion he thought the payment was worth every penny! I don't think I ever saw him laugh so much.

My father was eccentric and his need for attention, possibly the result of his own childhood, could have been part of the reason for my parent's incompatibility. His eccentricity might also explain why he chose a Heinkel for our first car. Dad's excuse for buying it was the petrol shortage, resulting from the Suez Crisis. Our neighbours had already bought the BMW Isetta for this reason.

These three-wheeled cars were known as 'bubble cars', because of their rounded shape. Ours was a dull, pale green colour. It didn't like steep hills; a pity because Plymouth has more than its fair share of these. Sometimes, when it didn't make it the first time, we would have to reverse and take another run at it. Children would run alongside the car laughing and shouting: 'Here comes the bubble car!'

It did have some advantages. We had the model with a sun-roof. If we were stopped at traffic lights, and my father couldn't see them changing, he would stand up in the car, and look out of the sun-roof. Other times, he would put his hand out through the sun-roof to signal left or right.

His eccentricity often put a strain on an already strained household, like the week we were suddenly invaded by what seemed like a huge number of Hare Krishna monks. My father had taken me to visit their temple, on a trip to London, and he had kindly offered them hospitality, should they ever be in Plymouth. And surprise! – they did come to Plymouth and they did take up his invitation.

He had a keen interest in politics, which was how we ended up on one holiday in Wales. Dad had seen an advert for a holiday bungalow in 'The Morning Star,' a socialist newspaper. We teased him about the fact that he had been a member of the Communist Party in his youth – we found his membership card in a cupboard in the lounge, when clearing it out to decorate. Dad was no longer a communist, or even a socialist, but he still had a keen interest in politics, and occasionally bought the newspaper. Other than politics, reading was his main hobby, followed by walking.

The bungalow was owned by 'Red Emma' (our nickname for her, on account of the newspaper). It was damp, and in the middle of a field of long grass with a resident goat. On the very first night, my mother took a dislike to the goat because it made such a noise that it kept us all awake. After a couple of nights she threatened to put a sock in its mouth. I must admit the idea did cause some amusement.

The long and short of the holiday was that a bungalow, in the middle of a field of long grass, was not ideal holiday accommodation for a couple of asthmatic children. We ended up in the local hospital. After a shot of adrenalin, oxygen and an overnight stay for us both, my mother decided not to take her two daughters back to the bungalow. She took us home and left my father to enjoy the holiday alone – well he had paid for it and wasn't about to leave!

I do have happy memories of my father, but he was not the sort of person who knew how to spend time with young children. Most of my happy memories are associated with my mid to late teens when I started to appreciate his interest in politics.

It was through his involvement in politics that I met Joe Grimmond, the Liberal Party Leader, at a party rally. Although very young, when this happened, I remember the moment well. He made quite an impression on me. I think it was something to do with the fatherly way in which he bent down to shake my hand. He had a warm smile and looked very kind.

Later, when I was considering pursuing a career in Law, my father took me to listen to a speech by Lord Hailsham, a former conservative Lord Chancellor. At last, he was able to share an interest with one of his children, and because of this I developed a different relationship to that which my sister had with him. My father and sister were always at loggerheads.

Through his love of politics, I was introduced to debate, and the enjoyment to be had in a lively exchange of ideas. I can think of many such exchanges with Alan, but never to more positive effect than in our work. Perhaps this is why a career in law appealed to me. However, it is only enjoyable when the participants understand the process, and provided the exchange doesn't become too personal and develop into a full-blown argument. Debating with Alan was enjoyable. We respected the other's opinion. We did not expect to agree on everything, but found discussion helpful, as a means of confirming or checking whether we needed to change our position or view.

A trip to Moscow with my father in 1972 – my first trip abroad – gave me my first exposure to the power of propaganda, and the danger of not having the full picture when formulating opinions. The Vietnam War was still going on. Until this trip, the reporting I had seen tended to favour the American side of the story. While we were waiting at the airport to come home, I watched the Russian newsreels being shown on a television in the departure lounge. I saw the terrible things the Americans were doing.

This excursion, and spending a good deal of my early life in the company of Quakers, may have given me my strong dislike of injustice – another reason for wanting to pursue a career in law. But it was not to be. Failing my law A-level, while at the same time doing very well in economics, changed the course of my career. I lost my place to study law at university. I could have continued via articles, but this would have meant remaining dependent on my father. By doing a degree I was able to obtain a grant. Business Studies included economics and law. It seemed a natural choice, while I made my mind up over what career I would follow. Failing law had left me uncertain. And looking back, it seems as if fate was already beginning to take its course.

My father's real downside was his use of money as a way of controlling his family. It was stifling for everyone, but most of all for my mother. I decided from a young age that I would always try to avoid being in the same position: what was his and what was my mother's was his, except that she didn't have anything. She wasn't able to have any money of her own, not until she started to work as a remedial dance teacher, at the same time helping with scriptwriting, for a religious pro- gramme, produced by the local television company.

Money was the cause of a lot of the friction in the family. I don't think it was the root of my parents' unhappiness, but it certainly didn't help. The underlying friction between my parents did not create a stable home environment. I was pleased to leave it whenever possible, often depositing myself on friends, in order to get away.

Without any money of her own, my mother believed our welfare was best taken care of by her staying with my father, no matter how un- happy she was. The marriage certificate became a ball and chain: my mother finally managed to make her escape, but long after her children had left home.

After my parents separated, when I was in my late twenties, I felt like the piggy in the middle of three opposing sides – my father, my mother and my sister. There had never been a strong bond between my sister and myself. This may have been because my parents were too wrapped up in their own problems to see the effect they had on the re- lationship between their two daughters, and the age difference between Fiona and me didn't help. Our family became fractured and it was against this background that I developed many of my feelings about marriage, family, children and divorce.

It was difficult not to blame my father for the break-up of our family, and being pulled in three separate directions meant something would eventually give. My father was the weakest link, and finally we became estranged, but not until 1998. About a year later, I changed my name to Wood. This represented the moment when I broke free. I changed my name by deed and at the same time adopted the married title. For reasons which will become clearer later, Alan and I were not able to get married, but using the married title was a way to avoid any need for explanation or embarrassment. For instance when sharing a bed in a hotel, I didn't want people to think he was sharing a bed with his daughter. His daughter was only a few years younger than me after all, so it was possible that people could think this. Alan was over the moon when I told him I wanted to change my name to his.

My father and I were not reunited until 2007, a few months before he died. I am grateful that it happened in time.

And so it was that I told my mother, but not my father.

My mother was helpful from the start. All her training as a nurse came to the fore. I could understand how, at one point in her career, before she married my father, she had been the youngest night nurse in the country.

I was still hoping that Alan didn't have MND. Until the diagnosis was confirmed we could still hope. Nevertheless, it seemed very likely that this was the cause of his symptoms. Hence, I agreed with Mum that the best thing would be to find out everything we could. She was methodical, practical and seemed to know exactly how to help. It was Mum who telephoned the MND Association, and asked them to send me their information pack.

If it was MND, we hoped to help ourselves as much as possible, to keep control over our lives. We also hoped to find ways to influence the nature and speed of the disease, and there seemed little benefit in putting these things off any longer. The fact that Mum did it for me helped me to make that first step. She held my hand. At the time, my prayer was very much 'Please God - if it is MND, make it slow but kind.' I wanted Alan to be around for as long as possible, but with a good quality of life.

I read all the literature that the MND Association sent. Amongst other things, it described what was known about the disease – not much – and gave some information on the kind of support one might need or be able to get. I hoped we wouldn't need any of it for a while yet, but it was useful to have the information there, standing by for future reference.

I read everything I could find on the subject. I read that some vitamin and food supplements might be beneficial, so I got Alan to take them. There was no hard evidence for any of it, but we were (that is, he was) prepared to try almost anything and everything. We might find that magic formula which would halt or slow the deterioration! Anything was possible. Unlike me, Alan had never been one for vitamins and mineral supplements. He took a multivitamin and that was all. However, now he was more than willing to take whatever might help. He did complain that he rattled! I looked at our diet, but didn't feel there was much we should change as we had always been reasonably careful about what we ate because of his heart problem. Alan also started to have massages and acupuncture. He found these helped improve the use and feeling in his hands, if only for a short time afterwards.

In the main, we went on trying to be normal. We could do little else until Alan had his appointment at King's College, London. Then we might get a better idea of what we were up against.

4 April 2004

Alan went to Saunton, in the West Country, for a few days' golf. It was an annual trip with a few mates. He always looked forward to it.

He loved golf. He had long held an ambition to play to a handicap of single figures, and achieved this in his retirement. Soon after he retired, he became Chairman of his golf club. He appreciated the opportunity to keep the grey cells going, and give back something to a club that had given him so much pleasure, and many good friends, over the years.

8 April 2004

Alan arrived home feeling rather low. He had realised, while he was away, that this was the last time he would be going on this trip. For the first time, he let me know what he felt. He said, 'some days I feel I will be able to cope, and others I feel so low, I just want to give up.' I understood exactly what he meant about coping, but for me it was from a different perspective. We would each have to cope in different ways. Although perhaps the only real difference was that my life would go on afterwards.

4 May 2004

We were both looking forward to three weeks away at the apartment in Spain. Neither of us had ever been to Cadiz, so we thought we would book a few days at the Parador there. We could drive there via the coastal route, and after our stay, take the route over the mountains back to the apartment.

It was an easy drive to Cadiz, and we walked a lot to see the tourist sites. In the evenings, we relaxed on the hotel terrace with a glass of wine before dinner, looking out over the Atlantic. After dinner, we sat on the same terrace drinking coffee and watching the sunset; the warm glow of the sun's rays spreading across the sky. As the sun disappeared below the distant horizon, where the ocean met the sky, it reminded me of a final curtain call – the final curtain call on a beautiful life.

Those few days in Cadiz were very special. We tried not to think of what the future held – wanting to make the most of now. The only thing that marred our stay was when Alan tripped up a step. We had been walking all day. Some passers-by helped me get him up. I could see he felt a bit of a fool. 'The step was in shadow, so he didn't see it,' I said, trying to make excuses for him.

His heart had been playing up since we arrived in Cadiz, and he had become more tired as the day went on, but neither of us could be sure that the fall was down to this. I didn't say anything, but I thought he wasn't picking his feet up properly. Added to him not being able to run – that time in St Moritz – and the spread of the fasciculations to other parts of his body, it was getting harder and harder to hope there might still be another explanation – something other than MND. Yet still we continued to hope against hope.

27 May 2004

Back at home.

In the night, Alan woke up and thought he felt a fasciculation in his chin. I had never asked him whether these were painful. I assumed they weren't, because he didn't notice them before the neurologist pointed them out, at that first appointment. It didn't occur to me to ask him what they felt like, but he must have felt them for it to have woken him up.

It scared us both, and we couldn't get back to sleep. I don't know what he was thinking. I didn't dare to ask him. I thought I could guess anyway, and didn't want his thoughts to confirm mine. We had talked about it, when we first found out he might have MND. It was our greatest fear – the fear that he would lose the ability to speak or breathe unaided.

2 June 2004

Alan had to have another EMG test at King's College, like the one he had had in December. I sat with him while they did the tests. I thought how brave he was. He said I didn't have to stay, but being there in the room with him while the test was done, meant I felt as though I was helping. If he had to go through it, the least I could do was be with him; and I had promised him we would be in this together.

The tests more or less confirmed that Alan had fasciculations everywhere, even in his tongue. The professor who was conducting the test, told us there and then. It was not the news we wanted to hear, but it was not unexpected.

6 June 2004

We went to the Summer Exhibition at the Royal Academy of Arts in Piccadilly, London, and had dinner afterwards at one of our favourite haunts – The Pavilion. It was at this restaurant that Alan, his son and I had had dinner all those years ago, when my 'yellow banana skin' exploded.

The 'yellow banana skin' was Alan's nickname for my yellow Capri. It was a very unlucky car. It was always breaking down, and on one occasion just managed to make it to the entrance of the smart hotel in Knightsbridge, where I was meeting Alan. It was exhaling blue smoke from its rear, as I pulled up. The doorman helped me to push it out of the way. He wasn't keen for my car to remain at the entrance, projecting completely the wrong image for the hotel!

So later, when it caught fire outside Alan's office close to Oxford Street, that was the end of it. We had been lucky to get out of the car just before it happened. The fire brigade arrived to put out the fire and we phoned the AA to come and tow away the burnt-out shell. While we waited for the AA, we had gone across to have dinner at The Pavilion and say 'goodbye' to a little piece of my motoring history.

We tried to keep going as usual. We still had no reason to think we wouldn't be able to live a normal life, and for some while yet. In fact, while we were having dinner, we thought that later in the year, it would be great to hold Alan's seventieth birthday bash at The Pavilion. We tended to prefer small private gatherings, and weren't usually party people. Dinner with a few friends was more our style. But Alan's seventieth was different, especially now.

10 June 2004

The appointment with the Professor at King's College, not the one that conducted the EMG, but the one who was the authority on MND, had come round. It felt like doomsday.

Our appointment was at 3.00 pm. We had made it later in the day, because it was impossible to know what the traffic would be like, and the hospital was not located in the best of places for us to get to. As we would discover when we got there, it is by no means a small hospital, a little intimidating in fact, and we still had to find our way to the department. But everything went smoothly, and we got to the appointment in plenty of time. We waited nervously in the large reception area. My heart sank, looking round at some of the other patients waiting with us. I hoped Alan wouldn't end up like them.

When we finally saw the Professor, he confirmed the diagnosis. It was not unexpected, but dashed completely any hopes that we had been able to allow ourselves. He looked at the test results, and asked Alan a few questions about the symptoms he was experiencing. Alan described his symptoms as follows:

> *'The strength in my shoulders is diminishing. When playing golf, I gradually lose the use of my right hand and 40/50% of my left. I am unable to hold the golf club with any strength, to undo the zip of my trousers or do up the belt or take money out of my change purse. My little finger has a mind of its own. The strength in the muscles controlling the thumbs is diminishing, so that turning keys becomes difficult or impossible. I feel a slight imbalance in my leg.'*

As he spoke these words, his voice in no way reflected the fear

49

he must have been feeling, the fear that the disease had already made significant inroads into his body and he was already losing control.

The Professor asked him to walk while he watched.

Although he confirmed that Alan had MND, he did offer us some encouragement. He seemed confident that Alan should be able to enjoy a good quality of life, and would still be moving around reasonably well, in two to three years' time. As the disease had started in his limbs, not his speech, Alan had the most common type known as Amyotrophic Lateral Sclerosis.* He went on to say there was a chance Alan would make his eightieth birthday.

The Professor's prognosis was good news in the scheme of things, and it helped us in another respect. We had been trying to work out how we would break the news to Michael and Caroline, Alan's son and daughter. At least we would be able to offer some good news, in amongst the bad.

Alan had already spoken to his wife, explaining what we knew. This would have been at about the same time I had told my mother. Whatever the outcome of our appointment at King's, it was unlikely to produce the outcome we wanted – a different reason for Alan's symptoms. So he felt he should tell her, to give her some time before he would have to talk to his son and daughter.

Alan and his wife Valerie had been separated for almost eight years when I met him. I don't know why they split up, other than that he had had an affair. I don't know why he had the affair, or why he didn't go back to her, especially as they remained separated and did not divorce. He always hoped Valerie would meet someone else and want a divorce, so I knew it was something he would have liked, but he would not be the one to push for it. Somehow, they had come to a compromise. It almost worked. But, as with all compromises there were also sacrifices.

We talked about almost everything, except what happened when he separated from his wife.

From my point of view, a piece of paper wasn't crucial – unless we had children. My own experience of my parents' marriage, and his experience, both confirmed to me that a marriage certificate was no guarantee of lasting love. In a happy relationship, it is a tangible expression of the special love between two people. I would have liked this and I think Alan would too.

The nearest we came to the subject of marriage was when his daughter told us she was expecting his first grandchild, in 1991. Until this point, Alan had always said he didn't want more children. I don't know why he felt this way, although I suspect it had something to do with the pain he had experienced at the time of his separation. I am sure there was a lot of pain for them all at that time. Caroline would have been about ten years old when her father left home. I would learn much later, in the last part of Alan's illness, that she had been hit particularly hard by it. Michael was two years younger and less aware. But any unhealed wounds were not readily apparent when I came on the scene.

I do know that Alan carried the guilt of the pain he caused. One of the reasons I loved him and admired him was because he never shirked his duties in anything. He was the most reliable person I have ever known. He had a strong sense of devotion to me, and to his children. He also had a strong sense of duty to his wife, as the mother of his children. I never discouraged it. In fact I did the opposite, and sometimes wonder if this increased his sense of guilt. In a way I was supporting her, and I am not sure this was right. But that is what I did, influenced by my own background.

Two weeks before Alan died, when I was driving him to the hospice – so I could have a respite day – I asked him why he had not divorced his wife. Why did I ask him then? For some reason, I needed to know the answer to this, now that his life was coming to an end. But why was it suddenly important to me? Effectively I was asking him why we had not married. I had been prepared to live like this all this time. It was too late to change things. So why did I ask then? I don't know, except that I was losing him and I felt insecure. What was I going to do without him?

He didn't answer me straight away.

Almost a week later, only a few days before he died, he said, 'she always let me see the children.' I had finally pushed, and I had finally got the answer to the question I had asked him. It must surely have been waiting in the recesses of his mind, for an appropriate moment to come out – expecting me to ask, but hoping I wouldn't. Now it didn't matter any more. He had always safeguarded his relationship with his children by not asking his wife for a divorce, and so we had never married, even though it was something we would both have liked very much. Caroline telling us that she was pregnant brought up the subject of children which had hung in the air between us for a long time. Now Alan asked me if I would like to have children. Until this point he had not wanted any more. I had wanted them. I had wanted a family, like the one I had longed for when I was growing up – dependable, providing unconditional love and a feeling of belonging. He was aware that I had wanted children. After all, I had given him enough hints. When we moved into our house, I had decorated the little bedroom to match my hopes. For a long time it was going to be the baby's room. He couldn't have failed to have noticed. But I never pushed the subject. I knew that he didn't want any more.

He had obviously been thinking for sometime, after we learnt Caroline's news, about what to say about his change of heart.

He chose the moment when I was sitting at the kitchen table –

doing some paperwork. Standing behind me, he put his arms around me. I could tell he was going to say something important, from the way he looked at me when he walked into the room. He hugged me tightly, and said, 'I think I would be happy about us having a child of our own, if it is still important to you; if you would still like children.'

Alan and I had become like two peas in a pod. Although I was more of a pea in his pod, it was always a very comfortable pod to be in. I had always felt safe and happy for all the time we had been together. Was this the moment when he finally felt safe in our relationship?

What he was suggesting was very tempting. It was possible as I was still only thirty-five, although he was fifty-seven. I would have leapt at it several years earlier. But now I was torn. Part of me did and part of me didn't want children. I needed to get accustomed to the possibility again, having shelved it for so long.

We didn't get any further, because I was diagnosed with a condition that made it difficult for me to conceive. If we had been able to have children, I would have pushed for marriage. Clearly, neither was meant to be.

It was better to be grateful for what we had. As a result, I was happy to let Alan's grandchildren and his family fill the gap left by my own family and an inability to have my own children. Besides, I had welcomed them into my life from the beginning, something that naturally made Alan very happy. It made us both very happy.

When his first grandchild, James was born in 1992, I discovered how much he loved children, especially babies. He couldn't wait to hold a baby in his arms. He held his grandson as he must have held his daughter that first time, as if a treasure too beautiful to ever let go.

So it was that he needed to be there for his daughter, when his baby grandson had meningitis. We took a small portable television into the hospital for Caroline and Reg, James's dad, to watch while they stayed with him. It hopefully gave them something to while away some of the hours. I still have the picture in my mind of James, being held by his father. They were both on the hospital bed, and there were tubes attached to James's tiny wrists. We had taken in a bottle of red wine to the hospital, to consume with some pizzas. Reg cradled his son in his left arm and held a glass of wine in his right hand. We left them like this, watching the football match on the television. Alan, Caroline and I went out to get the pizzas to take back to the hospital. It can't have been easy trying to follow the ball on the small television screen, but we hoped it would help pass the difficult days ahead.

My contact with Valerie was limited, probably not surprisingly, although I always thought we got on well under the circumstances. We saw each other on family occasions, such as Christmas. After the birth of James, we saw each other on not so special family occasions as well.

We all went to Euro Disney together in 1999. It was a special treat for James's birthday. I enjoyed the less adventurous rides with Alan's grandson, while all the other adults enjoyed the thrills of the scary rides. We had a great time.

Caroline and Michael would need Valerie's support. They were inevitably closer to their mother.

Now we had to find a way to tell them.

As luck would have it, Michael was coming over with his family, for a visit. He had gone to Australia to work and eventually emigrated. It was there, through his work, that he met his wife Stephanie – an English girl.

Michael went to Australia at the end of December 1987, to begin a career in the film industry. We were in Cornwall to celebrate New Year that year, so we drove to Gatwick airport and back again, all on the same day, to see him off. Alan took a bottle of champagne, in a wine cooler. We drank the champagne out of plastic cups – Caroline and Valerie were also there – before waving him on his way, through to departures. Alan and I kept all the corks from important celebrations in a drawer; including when Caroline told us she was expecting a baby. The cork from Michael's send-off, resides in the drawer with all the others.

After he emigrated, we went to Australia to see Michael, and latter on his family, a few times. The first time had been at the end of 1993, before he got married. We stopped off in Bangkok.

Thailand became a favourite stop-over on future trips because of its culture, people, beautiful temples and scenery. We loved the intricate detail of the golden temples. Their quiet calm provides a refuge from the busy activity of the water-buses and barges on the Chao Phya River, and an escape from the exhaust fumes and street noise of Bangkok.

A 'must' for each visit was dinner at The China House. The restaurant, in a two-storey colonial building, was close to the Oriental Hotel, which owned it. It reminded me, from the outside, of the buildings often featured in films about the Vietnam War. We always ordered the Peking Duck. The crispy outer layer was served first, carved at the table, and then the rest of the meat came later, as a separate dish.

On one stop-over, we took a taxi from Bangkok to the coastal resort of Hua Hin. We stayed in a luxurious hotel overlooking a long sandy beach, but I particularly remember the journey. As we left the city, the buildings gave way to rice fields and then further on, these were replaced by tropical plantations and lush vegetation dotted with wooden huts. It was quite different from any other place we had been.

On that first visit, we arrived in Sydney in time to celebrate New Year's Day with Michael and his then-girl-friend, Sam. We had lunch at a famous restaurant at Watson Bay, called Doyles. It was extremely hot, but nevertheless a glorious day. The sun beat down on the large umbrella above our table, which attempted to protect us while we enjoyed champagne and fish. Another champagne cork marks that occasion. The water lapped up the beach, not far from our table. New Year seemed an appropriate time for our first trip to Australia. And it was a perfect first day of the year.

The news of Alan's diagnosis was not the sort of news to announce over the phone, especially as this could be avoided. So we decided to wait until Michael arrived, and tell both of them at the same time.

12 June 2004

We went to a summer event at James's school, and enjoyed the Pimm's. It was strange: we had just had the death sentence confirmed, yet we were buoyant. We could be buoyant because it looked as though we still had a couple of years at least, with a reasonable quality of life.

The next day we went to Cornwall. The opportunity to tell Michael and Caroline would come when we got back from there.

We decided to tell only close family, for the time being. We wouldn't tell anyone else, including our friends in Cornwall. We would only let others know when we could no longer hide the effects of the disease.

Sometimes, when Alan played a friendly game of golf in Cornwall, I walked around with him. So it would not have seemed out of place for me to join him, as I did this time. He had given up playing in golf competitions – ever since those few days at Saunton – but still managed to play in friendly matches. Attaching a paper clip to his trouser zip enabled him to look after himself, if he got caught short. For the moment, we had solved one embarrassing problem. I went round with him in case he had any unexpected problems. This meant he could relax and enjoy the game. We could enjoy time together, and I would be there if he needed any help.

He started to become anxious that something would happen which he would not be able to deal with himself and I started to become anxious for him.

I pushed his electric trolley, to give me something to do, as I don't play. Brian, Alan's golfing buddy in Cornwall, told me that I needn't hold on all the time, once I had started it. 'If you let go, it will go so far, but then come to a halt,' he said. I decided to give it a try. Shortly after I let go, I realised the trolley wasn't going to stop! I ran up the fairway after it. By now it had made a good head start. If it hadn't toppled over the edge of a bunker at the top, and fallen in and died, I think I might still be chasing the damn thing round the course! They all wished that they had had a video camera, so they could have filmed me, and it caused much hilarity for the rest of the round, and at lunch afterwards.

21 June 2004

We returned home from Cornwall.

How do you tell the people you love that you have a cruel disease with no hope of a cure? I still don't know how Alan told me.

There was no reason to delay any longer, but telling them was going to be awful. We had agreed that we would start by telling them we had some difficult news, but it could be worse. Well it was better than the way we had first been given the news. I hope we were more sensitive than the neurologist who first came out with it to Alan.

For some reason we couldn't get Michael and Caroline together, to tell them. I think it was because we were going to Spain, and needed to tell them before we went. We ended up telling Caroline first. We told her that Alan had been diagnosed with a terminal illness, but that he did not have the worst type. The prognosis was good, in the sense that we appeared to have some time on our side. We told her what the Professor at King's had told us. The three of us ended up in a group hug; I am not sure who was consoling who.

Alan had to give Michael the news without me. I can't remember why I wasn't there. Alan told me how his son had cried and how difficult it had been to tell him. One of the reasons Michael and his family had made this trip was because they wanted to return to the UK permanently. They wanted to be nearer family, now they had two children, Tilly and Dexter. Their timing was fortuitous, but it was also cruel – they were coming back just as we had learnt that Alan had MND.

Still, it looked as though we would have some quality time with them all. We had reason to look forward with some hope.

Preparing for Battle

28 June 2004

Our trip to Spain was relaxing and enjoyable. Our spirits had been boosted by the better-than-expected forecast of the progression of Alan's illness. Since November we had been living on a knife-edge: knowing, but not knowing. Now we simply wanted to make the most of the time we had, before we would have to deal with the worst effects of the disease; and it seemed that we still had plenty of time before the stages of the disease we feared most. It looked as though Alan would still be able to be active and in control of his life for some time to come. Being active and self-reliant was very important to him.

Alan had always been a keen sportsman. As a young man, he enjoyed playing rugby, in spite of being injured continually in the game at school. His passion for sport came from his father, particularly his passion for cycling. Like his father, Alan took part in cycle racing in his youth, and he raced for the Polytechnic Cycling Club during the 1950's, before and after his National Service. He won numerous medals during these years, including Fastest Junior in 1951. He was always supported by his father, and whenever possible by his brother.

Alan toured all over the country to cycle race, and it was on one of these tours that he met his first love, Glenys. They wrote to each other while he was stationed in Egypt, in the Canal Zone, but she ended the relationship soon after he returned. She had let him know by letter, so he never saw her again. He kept the letter, and occasionally talked to me of her. It occurred to him that his life might have turned out very differently, if she had felt the same for him as he did for her. Fortunately, for me at least, she didn't.

The time Alan spent on National Service in Egypt allowed him to indulge in his love of sport. As with most things, he made the best of the situation; but still National Service couldn't have been much fun, especially as he narrowly escaped being killed. This happened while he was helping to protect their base, when it came under attack from Egyptian insurgents. An enemy bullet skimmed his arm. He was lying on the ground to avoid enemy fire, and luckily, just before the bullet hit him, he decided to turn over, thus avoiding a fatal wound.

But when not defending the base, he found plenty of opportunity to play rugby. He loved the game so much that he continued to play after he returned home, right up until he suffered a severe head injury. This happened when he was playing, on behalf of his employer, The Design Group, in an interagency match. The ball hit him with considerable force on the forehead, and had it been a couple of inches to the left or right, he might have lost the sight of one of his eyes. At times, during Alan's illness, I wondered if this had left a weakness – always searching for the trigger to the disease. Who knows?

He enjoyed watching sport as well. This was lucky because it was one of the few ways he could pass the long hours of the day towards the end of his life and still get some pleasure. He used to watch all kinds – rugby, cycling, cricket, football, boxing or tennis. You name it; he probably watched it. Sometimes he would make a comment, and the commentator would then say exactly the same thing. He always laughed when I told him he should have been a sports commentator, but it was true. He would have been good at it.

Sport was one of the interests he shared with his brother, Lionel. They had both gone to the 1948 Olympics when they were held in London, to watch the cycling and athletic events. I was reminded of this when I discovered his diaries. These were all in a trunk that Alan kept in the garage. The entry tickets from all those years ago were there! Just some of many mementos from his past.

One day, when I was helping him to clear out the garage, I uncovered the trunk. I didn't know it was there. The garage was very much

Alan's domain. I knelt down and opened it, not expecting to find anything important. Skimming the surface of its contents, I was surprised at what it contained. It made me look up at Alan, wondering why he had kept it in the garage for so long. I realised he wasn't looking at me, just staring into the contents of the trunk. He was deep in thought, and something told me he didn't feel like going through it. Something made me say, 'I think we had better leave this – perhaps another day.'

The opportunity to talk about the things in the trunk together passed us by.

I didn't open it again until nine months after he died. Like him, I had been putting it off. But it was his birthday, and I felt a sudden urge to be close to him. It was full of items from his life before we met; some of the pain of his life and also some of the joy. I wanted him to be there with me, to tell me the stories behind the things he had kept for so long, such as the fez from Cairo, or the letters and cards carefully wrapped in tissue, from the birth of his daughter. He had missed her birth because he was in hospital with pleurisy. He had often spoken of this. It was very apparent that he was upset that he was not around for this special event in his life. I suddenly realised that the last time he closed the lid down on this trunk must have been the time he put the lid on a lot of his life. He was not a man to dwell on the past – certainly the painful parts. 'Why dwell on something you cannot change?' he would have said.

But there were so many things I would have liked him to tell me about. After all, they had been important enough for him to want to keep them.

Amongst the various mementos, there were old school photographs and certificates. Alan was not academic. He went to St Olave's and St Saviour's Grammar School in London, and was quite happy when it was time to leave. Nevertheless, I know he appreciated the background it gave him. Apart from his family and attending church, it was where he learnt most of his values and strong sense of responsibility. He became an Old Olavian when he left, and was still an Old Olavian when he died. I remember being highly amused on the occasion when he stood in the living room, in front of my mother and me, and started to sing his old school song. With his arm across his chest, and hand on heart, he started to sing 'Olaf to raise the song, Olaf to bear along, Olaf to right the wrong till all our fight be fought ...'

The trunk contained the years that made the man I knew.

In all that time, he had enjoyed a great deal of control over his life, made possible through his business success which was owed to his love of a challenge, his reliability and his strong entrepreneurial skills. These skills first came to light while he was still at St Olave's. He used to gather unwanted comics from his friends, to sell on at school.

Alongside these factors, he was blessed with good fortune, until being diagnosed with MND that is. I think he stumbled into communication and design, rather than it being a conscious move, but his natural appreciation for design helped him to become successful in this field. Where this appreciation came from I have no idea. As he tended to take after his father, perhaps it was through him. That was probably where his love of music started, going to concerts together. But I am not aware of any shared appreciation for design. Alan, his brother and father all wrote a lot, so in this sense they were creative. They didn't just write letters to one another, when they were apart. They had poetry-writing competitions as well. The following poem accompanied a letter from his father, just before Alan returned from Egypt:

He'll wander round in civvy jacket

Causing quite a blessed racket

No symphony concerts will we hear

But Radio Luxemburg will blast our ear

As he often said during his illness, 'I have had a wonderful life', but the disease was gradually eroding the control that had made his life what it had been; one lived to the fullest. With that erosion went the motivation to overcome the challenges of the disease.

The final stages of MND are often likened to being locked in one's own body, unable to communicate or breathe unaided. Alan had never been interested in learning how to use a computer, although he could touch type, and he certainly didn't want to have to use one to communicate his needs. As far as he was concerned, should that be needed, he wouldn't want to go on living. If he couldn't speak it would mean he couldn't enjoy food either; the disease would have reached an intolerable stage.

While I knew Alan could type; it had been through the contents of the trunk that I discovered that he had acquired this skill in order to be a duty clerk, when he was doing his National Service. There had been a memo in the trunk that he must have typed to pass a particularly boring day in the office, while he was serving in Egypt:

From:-   Royal Air Force, Abu Sueir, MEAF 10

To:-   Headquarters No 205 Group, MEAF25

Abolition of Slavery

1 *Reference is made to East African Trading Post manuscript of the 10th instance.*

2 *It seems that Captain Blood finds it difficult to supply us with "new blood", so to speak, and he has written to us as to whether our allotment of thirty two and a half slaves per month can be decreased to, as he suggests, perhaps fifteen and a half.*

3 *After careful consideration of the manning required by this station, it is felt that a drop in slave labour can be shouldered by us, BUT a drop of seventeen is rather more than we bar gained for …*

Signed AW

But he lacked the inclination to learn to use a computer, something he had always happily delegated to me. He preferred to write using an attractive pen. Losing the use of his hands through MND would make this impossible, and much of his warmth, humour and sensitivity were apparent from his writing. It would be one of many losses.

He coped with almost everything the disease threw at him. He was amazing. But he dreaded losing the ability to speak or breathe unaided. At least while he could speak, he could instantly communicate his needs.

Machines can help. The computer software used by the well-known physicist Stephen Hawking, an MND sufferer, is one method. It does require effort and determination especially for someone like Alan who had not used computers in his everyday life, but many people with MND find it a valuable aid to communication. It comes with a few commonly used words and phrases but mostly each word has to be inputted, so it requires patience. Gradually, though one can build up ones own personalised vocabulary.

In Alan's case, he had had 'a wonderful life' and he didn't want to live with the worst stages of MND. He didn't have the motivation that others might have. But then Alan had always been physically active. Simply having the use of his brain, while being completely dependent on others in the worst stages of the disease, would not be enough to motivate him. In fact it would become intolerable for him.

And Alan had made it clear, at a very early stage, that when the disease became intolerable for him, he would want to go to Switzerland, to Dignitas. He wanted to be allowed to die at the time of his choosing, just as Diane Pretty had wanted. He could not be assisted to do this in the UK, but he could in Switzerland. Dignitas is an organisation which helps people to carry out their wishes. It was all discussed with his daughter and son and he knew he had all our support. However, as time went by, his early decision would prove easier said than done.

I suppose it should have been apparent, at this point, that we might not have had the time we imagined. Perhaps we should have guessed it from the changes that had already occurred. After all, Alan had described, at his appointment with the Professor, that he had lost the use of forty to fifty percent of his left hand and some of the use of his right while playing a game of golf. He was already having some minor problems with his legs, as we had experienced in St Moritz.

However, we preferred to accept what we had been told, and assumed the need to go to Switzerland would be some way off. For the moment, it was important to enjoy what time we had, and try to find ways to fend off the disease.

In Spain, Alan's hands seemed better, just as they had been the previous time. We weren't sure, however, whether this was because of the warm climate, or because he had started to take a drug called riluzole*. It was recommended that he should start taking it as soon as possible, when he had been formally diagnosed in June because it was thought to slow the disease. We hoped it was having some effect.

But while we were in Spain, Alan found that he could no longer do power walks along the beach. His legs became tired easily. It was difficult not to be disheartened by this change. He must have wondered if the prognosis was correct because of the changes he was experiencing, but we wanted to believe it. We wanted to believe we had time with a reasonable quality of life. After all, we had been told there was a good chance Alan would see not only his seventieth, but his eightieth birthday as well.

I held on to this, blind to what was happening in front of me. It was like this for me until the end, although I don't think it was for Alan. Obviously, he would have been much more aware of the deterioration, and when I think back, there were many times when he tried to warn me that the end was closer than I thought.

6 July 2004

We arrived home from Spain to find a lovely note of support from Caroline. The note said that if we needed any help we only had to ask. We were both moved by it.

In reality, it would be very difficult to burden our close relatives or friends with our difficulties. They had their own lives and problems, and unless specific help was offered, we tended to try to cope. Besides it wasn't an easy thing to ask, because we had always been a very private and self-contained couple. As the disease ran its course though, self-reliance became a necessity rather than a choice more often than not, and it came at enormous emotional cost to us both.

We did feel we should be able to ask for and rely on help from medical and various other professionals, whose job it was to support us. However, when I did ask or made it apparent that I needed assistance, it was often not forthcoming; when it did come, it was usually too late.

When you are screaming down the telephone, because you haven't been able to get the support you need to do the job you want to do, you would think the person on the other end of the phone would guess that you are on the very edge! I am sure they wanted to help, and were simply up against their own problems, but sometimes just a bit of information or action early enough, would have made all the difference.

In these very early stages of the disease, there was little that could be done except collect information for later, and try to be prepared. I had some experience of the equipment we might need, from my limited time of looking after Sarah. However, knowing everything there was to know about all the types of assistance available, and how to get it, would turn out to be a completely different matter. Eventually, I would need a lot of advice from the medical profession and social services. It would have been so helpful at this stage to have had comprehensive information about what was ahead of us, what help we could expect and what we should already be considering.

There were, however, many people who were willing to tell us what they thought we should do. Sadly, I am not referring here to professional advice. I am referring to those who felt they knew best! I suppose they meant well, but how would they have taken it had they been in our shoes? Strongly worded advice often comes over as criticism just when you least need it; it still amazes me that people can do that. One person, a woman Alan went to for a massage, specialised in this kind of advice. She had been recommended to us, and when Alan went along to her, I would drive him, because her clinic was some way away, and she felt he would get more benefit if he didn't drive immediately afterwards. But then I would find when I went in with him, that I was being quizzed about his diet. She told me that it was likely Alan was intolerant of many of the foods I was feeding him; that they were poisonous to his system. I am sure she intended to be helpful, but nevertheless it was insensitive. For a while, I was open-minded, and prepared to go along with it. It was worth considering anything.

Although I felt we had generally been good about diet, I had been trying for a couple of years to get Alan to go to a nutritionist. This was because he had never seemed to completely recover from a virus that hit him on the way back from Scotland in 2001.

I had flown to Inverness to join him for a few days, at the end of the annual Golf Open. We were staying overnight in the Lake District, to break the journey home. Alan went down with the virus over dinner. We had been waiting for a long time for our dinner. Within moments of finally sitting down to our meal, he wanted to leave the table. He said, 'I don't feel like eating this I am afraid, Angel. I just want to go to the room. You stay and eat yours.' I ate dinner alone, and didn't realise just how ill he was. I thought he had lost his appetite through waiting so long, and because he was tired.

But all night he was very unwell. When we left the next day, we had to stop for some petrol. Alan filled the car up, and asked me to pay. I had just got out of the car when he told me to take over filling it up. I did so, and the next thing I saw was him keeling over. He was by the pay kiosk. I didn't know if he had fallen into the wall and hit his head, or if he had had a heart attack. He wasn't moving. I remember replacing the nozzle of the petrol pump and running over to him. All the time I was yelling: 'Alan, Alan.'. I knelt down, lifted his head, and held it in my lap. I was distraught. I thought I had lost him – he wasn't answering me. A little girl, who had come over to us while I was holding him, was sitting in front of me. She was trying to comfort me – her eyes reflecting my sense of utter desperation. It seemed like an age before he came round. I think the little girl and I were both praying. She stayed with me, while the garage called for an ambulance. They took Alan to the hospital in Kendal. I followed in the car. It was decided that it was not a heart attack; it was the effect of the virus. Alan had always had a very poor immune system. He would acquire any infection going, ever since the age of two, when he was taken to hospital with a high temperature and a swelling on his neck. The cause was not explained. The swelling was lanced and his temperature went back to normal. Thank goodness for the discovery of penicillin in 1928, before he was born!

Anyway, I wondered if he was lacking in some essential vitamin or mineral or perhaps his hormones were out of balance. It could just as easily have been his age, but I thought it worth checking and taking Alan to a nutritionist. Then the neurologist's tests had proved that all his vitamin levels were acceptable, so it went on a back burner. But perhaps they had missed something. Perhaps there was something in the advice the masseuse kept giving me?

Alan wasn't against her advice, up to a point. We did adopt some of her suggestions, if only in the vague hope that it might slow the progression of the disease. However, it was more important to him, now that he had been diagnosed, to eat what he enjoyed for as long as he was able.

One of the things she suggested was bathing in mineral salts. If nothing else, this was pleasurable to do, so Alan was very happy to take this on board. But overall the constant advice became increasingly wearing, and to avoid a lecture I stopped going in with him. I did my weekly food shop while he had his massage. Afterwards, I waited in the car.

On what turned out to be our last visit though, I had to go in to the appointment with Alan, because he needed help. She used the opportunity to start on me again. Why couldn't she just leave me alone! I really didn't need to be told that I was effectively the cause of his disease or, as she put it, I 'was poisoning him.' It was a cruel thing to say. I was simply trying to do my best in an impossible situation.

There were so many things that might have caused Alan to get MND. Believe me, I have never stopped wondering whether had we done this or not done that, we might have avoided the disease. But for all I know, the diet we adopted for Alan's heart could have been responsible for delaying the onset of MND.

I had flu at the time and was feeling very down. Her attack left me in tears and I drove all the way home in this state. After we got home, I told Alan I couldn't take him again. We would have to find someone else to give him his massage.

In the end we would not have been able to go to the 'Poison Dwarf', as we had started to call her, for much longer. Alan would not have been able to negotiate the staircase to her treatment room. Thankfully, we found someone else who was prepared to come to the house, and this worked out much better all round.

Another remark that I seemed to hear quite frequently, and found upsetting, was: 'well, that's what you do for the people you love.' In the voice I sensed, 'you just have to get on with it.' It wasn't said with any understanding. It was said in a way that suggested they couldn't really have cared.

I felt like saying: 'you try it then!' It is what you do for people you love, but that doesn't make it easy, in fact it makes it much harder. Then there were the times when I just didn't feel like it. Did that mean I didn't love Alan? Something to add to a whole list of guilt feelings the disease caused me to accumulate over time.

Life went on pretty much as usual for some time. In the main, when we hit a problem, we were able to deal with it reasonably easily, at least at the physical level. Emotionally, it was quite different. Each time Alan couldn't do something else it affected us both. We both felt low. However, we tended to keep it to ourselves, each wanting to appear positive for the other.

He started to find it virtually impossible to turn small keys, such as the one to unlock the front door, or the one to turn on the car ignition. However, he invented a way to overcome the problem. By sticking pieces of rubber to either side of the inside edges of a pair of pliers, he was able to use these to grip keys and turn them. For a while he got a kick out of mastering difficulties on his own. He still had control. He was still independent. He carried the pliers around in his pocket, and it is probably a good job he wasn't stopped by the police, and asked to explain why he kept a pair of pliers with him!

He avoided shirts with buttons, unless the occasion demanded one. If it did, then he had to ask me to do the buttons, and his tie. He disliked having to ask. He started to wear slip on shoes, rather than those with laces. He loved shoes, but now wore only those he could put on easily himself.

Appearance was still important, and remained so virtually to the end. It demonstrated his determination not to give in to the disease, and maintain some control, albeit negligible.

8 July 2004

We had an appointment to see Alan's consultant cardiologist. A change from seeing a consultant for MND! Alan was experiencing an ever-increasing incidence of heart fibrillation and flutter. He was getting tired more easily, and we didn't know how much of this to put down to the MND. We also thought that his heart condition could be putting an additional strain on his system, with the potential to speed up the course of the MND. Hence we wanted to try to solve it. In any case, dealing with MND was going to be quite enough.

I didn't take to Alan's cardiologist. We hadn't met before. Nowadays, Alan and I went to all his appointments together. After all, I had promised we would be 'in this together.' I don't think he took to me either. He was one of those members of the medical profession who conveyed the opinion that they always know best. You shouldn't need to query their advice. However, we did. Neither of us had complete confidence in him now. We had been through a lot – enough to start to ask questions.

In July the previous year, when we were away on what should have been a wonderful cruise, Alan's heart condition became more problematic It started in Istanbul, a place I had long wanted to visit; a place which appealed to us both for all sorts of reasons. Neither Alan nor I went to church except for Midnight Mass at Christmas and weddings and funerals. We were not, what you might call, religious. However, I think we would both have said that we believed in something, even if it can't be explained. My introduction to religion had been to go to a Quaker Sunday School. Then my mother reverted to Methodism, my father became a Unitarian, and I went to a Church of England school. Alan described himself as agnostic, and it wasn't until the Thursday before he died that I discovered he attended a Congregationalist church as a boy. We were at the Royal Brompton Hospital for a sleep test to check on his oxygen levels. One of the questions on the admission form, asked for his religion. I said 'What shall I put?' He had always said 'Put Church of England' or 'Christian', when I had asked him before. I don't really know why I didn't put one of these, but something made me ask again. He said 'Congregationalist'. I looked from the form to him, and he must have registered my surprise – I had never known, not in all the years we had been together, This turned out to be just a few days before he died, and I think it suddenly became important to him that it should be right.

So, although not outwardly religious, deep down we each had our reasons to be interested in religion. We were also interested in the influence of religion on peoples and cultures, and in this respect Istanbul had plenty to offer, with its mixture of Asian and European cultures, Christianity and Islam, and also the evidence, all round the city, of the once great power of the Ottomans.

We spent a couple of days there, before joining the cruise ship, and loved it. We enjoyed weaving our way round the fascinating labyrinth of little shops of the Grand Bazaar, which sold everything and anything, and the challenge of trying to pre-empt overcharging by the taxi drivers. We stood in awe in the great Blue Mosque with its interior virtually covered in blue tile-work. We visited the Haghia Sofia, which was designed as an earthly mirror of the heavens. It still imparted some of that celestial feeling in its glistening mosaics, having been a church, then a mosque, and then, finally a museum.

We couldn't leave Istanbul without a visit to the Topkapi Palace, to see the famous Topkapi dagger – the star in that Peter Ustinov classic film. Studded with three giant emeralds; it was beautiful.

From the terrace of our hotel we could see across the Bosphorus to the city beyond. I couldn't help thinking that Istanbul had a great deal in common with Venice, which we had been to many years previously. They share spectacular architecture, by virtue of their once great trading history, and are both romantic cities to visit. We loved Istanbul so much that we kept saying to each other, 'we must come back here again', not realising that the time to do that would be stolen from us, not by Alan's heart condition, but something much more vicious.

Almost as soon as we boarded the ship, Alan's heart started to misbehave. It was a particularly bad attack of fast and irregular heart-beat. It was the first bad attack since he had been given cardioversion* earlier in the year in an attempt to cure the problem. Clearly it hadn't worked. What should have been a special holiday was spoiled, although he tried not to let it happen. This upset him a great deal, because he booked the cruise mainly for me. Other than winter holidays, most of our trips had been further afield, to South Africa and South America and to countries such as New Zealand and, of course, Australia. For a long time, I had been saying there were places closer to home I would like to see with him.

But from Istanbul, through the Bosphorus to Kusadasi and the great archaeological site of Ephesus, on to the Greek island of Santorini with its black volcanic sand, and then the Island of Stromboli north of Sicily, Alan's heart kept on beating at a fast and irregular rate. At one point the ship's doctor threatened to helicopter Alan to a hospital on the Italian mainland, but we persuaded him not to. We managed to reassure him that Alan's condition was not life-threatening. I hoped we were right.

The most romantic part of the trip, and the part I was particularly looking forward to, was sailing past the Stromboli volcano. We were scheduled to sail past it at midnight. But, it didn't happen as I had hoped. Alan was so tired from the heart problem that he fell asleep on the bed in the cabin, before we arrived. I went up on deck alone. It didn't feel romantic. I actually felt quite sad. I was too worried to wake Alan so we could share this moment, as I had planned. I had imagined I would feel his arms around me, as we watched the red hot lava spew from the crater, roll down the black sides of the volcano and fizzle into the sea directly below. While it was warm up on deck, close to the hot lava, I felt cold. The thought, that this was what life would be like without him, passed through my mind, like a ghost of the future.

We sailed on to Sorrento and 'did' the Amalfi coast. We visited Pompeii, but how Alan walked around there in the heat, with his heart problem, I will never know. He was determined to come with me, and share my enjoyment.

Our last-but-one stop was Portofino, where Alan's heart rhythm finally corrected itself. The doctor was relieved, but not as relieved as we were. He wondered why Alan hadn't been offered a pacemaker, instead of suffering for so many years. The medication he was taking clearly wasn't controlling the problem.

So we couldn't just sit in this cardiologist's consulting room and take his advice unquestioningly, especially now that Alan had MND as well. We asked a stream of questions. Amongst the questions was whether the heart problem, or the medication Alan had taken for years, could have contributed to the disease? We had to ask this; all the time looking for what might have triggered the disease. I suppose I thought that if there was a clue, there might be a chance of finding a way to halt or reverse it. But there wasn't any evidence.

We made it clear, in no uncertain terms, that life had to be made as easy as possible from this moment on. Everything had to be done to ensure that Alan's quality of life was as good as it could be, for as long as possible. His heart problem wasn't helping. It had never helped. The cardiologist could see it in my eyes. I was giving him a determined, even desperate look, which said I was relying on him to do something.

He agreed to do all he could, and to talk to his team about the possibilities. They would keep an open mind as to whether medication was still the best solution, especially now that Alan was taking riluzole. This was something the Professor at King's College had raised.

11 July 2004

Alan drove to Scotland, for the Golf Open at Troon. He was meeting Cyril, his golfing pal. They had been going to this annual event together for years. They had been a part of a group of 'lads', but over the years the group had dwindled. Only Alan and Cyril still went.

Alan looked forward to it every year. However, this trip would serve to highlight the level of deterioration.

Alan was not the sort of person to get depressed, but I could tell from his telephone calls, that he was at the very least, exceptionally low.

He telephoned me when he arrived, to let me know he had got there safely, and sounded a little upset. It transpired that he had been let down over his booking for an en-suite room. Some earlier arrivals were allocated his room. It got worse. His room was at the top of a steep narrow stairway with the bathroom downstairs. He could still manage stairs, provided he could take them slowly. He was clearly worried that he might get caught short in the night, and not be able to make it down the stairs to the bathroom in time.

I found myself asking 'Is there a sink in the room?' I would never have suggested such a thing before. But needs must, and he had been let down. It was not his fault. 'No' he said, 'but there is a window'. 'Is there anything outside?' I asked. 'No, just some bushes,' he replied. 'Well that's it – pee out of the window, if you have to!' God, I thought, is this me talking?

At that point, I wished I could have been there with him. My confident man sounded so vulnerable. I wanted to put my arms around him and tell him it was alright; I wanted to be there and to envelop him in my protective cloak, just as he had always done for me. Our roles were starting to reverse. They could never reverse completely though. He had always been my protector. In many ways he still is. He did all he could to try to keep me safe, even after he died.

We had always been happy in each other's company, but we also knew when to give the other space. Now we just wanted to be together. This trip made it evident. It would be the last time, other than respite or hospital that we would be apart for any length of time, and we would never be happy about it when we were.

When he phoned me again, I asked him how he was getting on with the bathroom. 'Fine' he said. I noted a little amusement in his voice. 'But the bushes below the window have taken a turn for the worse!' He managed a rather naughty laugh, and made me laugh with him.

Well it wasn't his fault. Furthermore, I was cross with the people who ran the bed and breakfast – for putting him through this. If they had kept their side of the bargain, he wouldn't have needed to resort to such measures! He would not have been caused unnecessary anxiety – anxiety that inevitably affected his heart.

The progress of the disease prevented him from taking time out from the Open to play golf with Cyril, as they had done in the past. On the bright side, they still managed to indulge in their joint love of good food and wine. The Poison Dwarf would not have approved!

But it was impossible for Alan not to compare what he could do now with what he could do a year ago, or even three months ago. It depressed him; he had to think about how far he walked, and where. In the past Alan would walk wherever and whenever possible. He preferred to take the stairs for exercise, rather than take a lift. Now he took the lift.

He tried to remain upbeat. He was still able to do a lot, but his confidence was already starting to be eroded by the disease.

Whether it was the anxiety or the riluzole we weren't sure, but Alan began to develop what was later diagnosed as irritable bowel syndrome (IBS). We had first noticed the symptoms in Spain, soon after Alan started to take the drug, so we were inclined to think it might be the cause. The problem recurred in Scotland, which wasn't helpful given the bathroom arrangements. In fact the bathroom arrangements may have been responsible, because they made him anxious.

19 July 2004

I flew to Glasgow to join Alan at the end of the Open; so we could spend a few days in Scotland, just as I had done in 2001 when he went down with the virus on our way back. We were booked into the same hotel that we had stayed in before. It was by Loch Torridon, but this time our stay was disappointing.

The previous time we had enjoyed it very much, which was why we wanted to go back there. The hotel organised activities that we hadn't tried before. The last time I had made an attempt at clay pigeon shooting. I had found the gun very heavy, because it was designed for a man, which was fine for Alan. I remember how the rebound of the gun, after pulling the trigger, gave me a bit of a painful shoulder the next day. But it wasn't enough to stop me wanting to do it again, provided I had a more appropriate gun. They had promised they would have one suitable for me the next time we came. But because Alan couldn't join me now, owing to the weakness in his hands and arms, I decided to give it a miss. The hotel was in a lovely spot by the lake, and we could still walk a little way round it after dinner, much as before, so all was not lost.

The weather was mixed, but it had been the last time. In a way this added to the magic of the scenery. On one of the days we were driving along in dense fog. Suddenly we came out of it to find the sun shining across a huge lake. On the other side was a mountain. It reminded me of Dartmoor, only it was even more beautiful.

So there wasn't anything specific to make our stay disappointing, except that this time we needed to take everything much more easily. It simply wasn't the same.

We decided to stay in Edinburgh for a couple of nights after that and we enjoyed our time there, perhaps because we didn't have anything to compare it with. The hotel was very comfortable, and we used the hop on/hop off tourist bus to see some of the sights. Alan didn't have any problem coping with it. Walking long distances was perceptibly more of an effort, but, for the most part, it didn't interfere with what we wanted to do together. Alan did let me do the shops alone!

The only thing which was the same, was Alan being unwell on the way back. This time it was the usual problem: his heart.

26 July 2004

We had an appointment with Alan's neurologist – an update following the full diagnosis at King's College, London.

After shaking hands with him, and making our polite introductions, we all sat down. The neurologist had the letter from King's with the diagnosis in his hand, and wanted to know how Alan was, and what changes had occurred since our last visit in March.

Alan mentioned the problem that had started in Spain, after taking riluzole – the one that was later diagnosed as IBS. He wondered whether it might be a side effect of the drug. However, it wasn't known to be. Alternatively, he wondered whether it was reacting negatively with his heart medication. The neurologist noted that we were waiting for the outcome of the cardiologist's deliberations, and suggested that Alan stop taking riluzole until then. He stopped, and didn't restart, as he was not sufficiently convinced of the benefits in his case. We will never know whether this was the right thing to do; perhaps the drug would have given us more time, but importantly, it was Alan's decision.

For the most part we asked questions about what we could be doing to prepare for the effects of the disease. It was felt that anything we needed could be handled locally. This would avoid going to King's. We could still go there for assessment and advice if we wanted to, but it was such a trek that we preferred to avoid this option, if possible. The minuses outweighed the pluses, at least as far as we could see. We decided it would be beneficial to continue to see this local neurologist privately, roughly every three months. He told us it wouldn't make any difference to the standard of care, if we saw him via the NHS. It was our choice, because we felt it was likely to be easier to access appointments quickly, should Alan's condition change suddenly.

One of the things we were told was that there isn't such a thing as remission. It might appear as though there is, because there could be long periods without any noticeable difference. However, all the time the disease would still be having an effect on the body. Something would happen – like walking along on a plateau for some time, and not seeing the edge. Suddenly you find you have walked over it. You have fallen to the next level, and there is no way to claw yourself back. Each level would represent a further deterioration, and bring Alan closer to the end of his life.

There was another reason for staying private. We felt we would be more likely to see the same neurologist each time, and continuity would allow changes to be more readily noticed. These were small ways in which we could try to maintain control, and hopefully help ourselves to adapt quickly to each level of change. In practice this would be easier said than done. The disease had its own agenda.

We tried not to bury our heads in the sand. We talked with the consultant about practical issues, such as adaptations we would need to organise for the house, and he told us an occupational therapist would be able to advise us. He suggested we visit our local hospice and see what support they could offer. Alan wasn't keen to go to the hospice. Apart from enabling me to have respite, and as a means to being supported at home, he never would be. He had his own plans.

As far as he was concerned, when the disease became too much, he would be going to Switzerland to die. Naturally, I wanted him to be around for as long as possible, but it was his life, his decision. I would lose him at some point to the disease. I had no right to stand in the way of what he needed to do. Besides, I loved him too much to watch him suffer. I simply wanted to make him as comfortable as possible at home for as long as he wanted to live. No one seemed to be able to make this any easier for me. However, as I would discover, they could make it an awful lot harder. Even Alan didn't always see the point in some of the things I wanted to do. Because he had his own plans, he was only really interested in what might delay or slow the disease.

It was in this vein, that the consultant recommended physiotherapy, and put us in touch with a private physiotherapist. Alan began to have a one-hour-long session every week, almost straight away, with a view to maintaining his mobility for as long as possible. He could still do the twenty minute exercise regime he had developed and done every morning - ever since I had known him. One of the exercises was press-ups. He used to raise himself up on his fingertips, but he couldn't do this any longer. In fact, I remember joking with him that I wasn't surprised he was losing the sensation in the ends of his fingers – wouldn't anyone, if they had been doing press-ups this way, for so many years!

When he showed the physiotherapist the exercises, she was genuinely impressed at what he could still do - for his age, let alone the fact that he had MND! However, she recommended ways to tailor them, so he would not overexert the muscles. He started using weights (dumbbells), to try to maintain the strength in his arms. He had soft balls to squeeze and 'Therapy Putty' to roll and manipulate, to try to maintain the flexibility in his fingers.

The neurologist wrote to Alan's GP following our appointment, recommending what he felt was necessary to get the wheels in motion, for later. What wheels, I ask myself now? There were so few, and none attached to any well-oiled machinery.

Assistance through our GP was covered by the NHS, as far as it was available. The GP notified the local hospice, which assigned a Macmillan nurse. She came to talk to us. If we needed anything, I just had to call. In time, I would learn that it wasn't that easy. Many staff worked part-time and consistency was a real problem. I can remember moments of sheer desperation when getting an answer machine. Only once did I resort to leaving a message. After all, what can an answer machine do when you need help now – later was often too late. A physiotherapist and occupational therapist also came from the hospice, to give us some initial advice. Regular contact was established with the district nurse from our surgery. She liaised with the GP, over those needs that they could directly influence – not many. However, they did apply for Attendance Allowance* on our behalf, and also enabled Alan to apply to, and be accepted by, our local council for the Blue Badge parking scheme.

At the beginning, it seemed we were getting enough support, but that was because we didn't need much at that point, and preferred to do things for ourselves, while we could. In reality, there wasn't a properly coordinated approach to the physical effects of the disease. Such an approach from an early stage, with increasing help as the disease inevitably made life more and more difficult, would have spared a lot of frustration and despair. The frustration and despair, caused by a complete lack of joined up-thinking and action, served to make the emotional difficulties of living with the disease, even harder.

We could not fault the dedication of those sent to try to help us. They spent many hours listening to our problems. However, more often than not, they were powerless to offer any practical assistance. Budgets were often given as the reason, although sometimes they simply lacked the correct information or any information at all.

In my view, in order to make a better death from MND, or other similar condition for both the sufferer and the people closest to them a key worker should be assigned, from the moment the disease is confirmed. Ideally, they would be part of, and supported by, a palliative care team in every major hospital. They would be responsible for liaising between all those involved in end-of-life care, such as the consultant, the GP, the district nurse, the local hospice and social services. The key worker would be trained to have a comprehensive knowledge of all the relevant support, and be in a position to access that support as soon as it is needed. In some regions this quality of care may be provided but it was not at all the case for us.

Initially, it may just be a case of monitoring. However, in so doing, they would be in a position to determine the speed of the disease, and at what stage the different types of support should be made available – funded or self-funded. They need to be able to discuss, give advice and coordinate the care package for the person suffering from MND at the various stages of the disease. Their sole objective should be to maintain as much control for the sufferer as possible – over their life, and eventually their death.

So often, I discovered some area of support via serendipity, and then had to make it happen through sheer determination. More frustratingly, I would find out about some area of support after the event, which could have made all the difference to my emotional and physical reserves. This would have left me less distraught, and more able to cope.

There aren't any drugs proven to effectively slow, let alone cure

MND, unlike some illnesses. It is likely to be a long time before there is. The only real help that can be offered is palliative care.

There doesn't seem to be a well-coordinated palliative care structure, for people suffering from MND, as there is with other terminal diseases, such as cancer. Some hospices have a difficulty taking MND patients, owing to the high level of care they require. Yet I would be left to look after Alan alone for most of the day. However, I was luckier than others, because our local hospice did take Alan for respite. But we still had to fight every inch of the way for the support we had, and I didn't feel I could rely on the hospice to take Alan when I needed the respite. If they didn't have the beds or the staff they couldn't take him.

And, even though we were prepared to pay for help, we couldn't get the advice or information, when we needed it! All this was in addition to dealing with the physical and emotional effect of the disease. The system that would not help Alan to die –when there was no hope, and he was in sufficient distress from the disease to no longer want to live – would not give him the support he needed, while he waited to die.

It was nearly always my own determination – mine, because Alan became too helpless – that made anything happen. No, it was not a good death. It will haunt me for the rest of my days.

For the moment, we wanted to keep life as normal as possible, and we were coping, at least on the physical level. For the time being, the lack of any coordinated approach did not occur to me. It did not occur to me until much later. In fact, it didn't occur to me until it started to happen in the very last stage of Alan's life. It was only then that I realised what a difference it would have made – too late.

9 August 2004

We were meant to be travelling to Cornwall, but had to delay our trip by a further day, to attend the funeral of Alan's aunt. We had already delayed our trip to say goodbye to Alan's son and his family. They ended up staying longer than planned, attempting to do as much preparation as possible, for their trial move back to the UK. But for the moment they had to return to Australia. Their extended stay was an unexpected bonus for us.

Alan decided to tell his brother about his illness, just before the funeral, so the family could be made aware. I am not sure if they would have noticed the change in Alan, but it seemed best to let his brother know so he could, in turn, tell their cousins, in particular Rosie and Joan, who Alan had been so close to, when they were all children.

The sun shone on the day of the funeral, as it would for Alan's. While we sat in the small chapel for the service, I couldn't help but wonder how long Alan and I had. Hopefully, quite a while yet, from what we had been told.

19 August 2004

There was a Test Match at the Oval. Alan and his brother organised to meet up on one of the days, to watch it. Apart from finding the steps in the underground station more difficult to negotiate on his own, he had a good day out. The only times I had been to a cricket match with him, we had taken a Fortnum and Mason's hamper and I read a book. He really preferred to go with someone who would appreciate the game!

1 September 2004

This was the day we had an appointment with the electrocardiologist. Another medical appointment! We bounced between these and trips to Cornwall and Spain. At least we could still make such trips.

It seems the cardiologist had finally come to the conclusion that, under the circumstances, a pacemaker would be the best solution. It had proved impossible to find out what interactions could occur between the heart medication and riluzole. This was due to the lack of data on people who suffered from both MND and Alan's heart condition. Alan was unique, but in this case it was not a benefit! It was hoped –we hoped –a pacemaker would improve his quality of life for a little longer, and at the very least, help him to cope better with MND.

I am not sure whether I have any regrets. Can you regret things that you cannot control? However, I do wish Alan had been offered a pacemaker a few years earlier. I am sure he wished the same. It would have made life before MND even better.

On the way to the appointment, it occurred to me that we had completely missed the Proms season. Normally, at this time of the year, we would be going to London for a concert. We had been every year, ever since I could remember.

I don't think there can be another music festival in the world like it. Where else would you hear the same exchanges between the Arena and Gallery audiences? As the piano is moved into position on the stage, the Arena shouts 'Heave' and the Gallery responds 'Ho,' and the rest of the audience laughs at the traditional banter between the two groups. At the end of the concert, the hall reverberates with the stomping of feet. It begins slowly, then becomes faster and faster, and louder and louder, until the conductor gives in, and comes back on stage to a huge cheer from the audience.

Attending a last night of the Proms is like nothing else. As the whole audience sings "Rule, Britannia", it is so funny watching the different nationalities, oblivious to the words, waving the flags of their own countries. Then the rousing finale as everyone stands to sing "Land of Hope and Glory." The emotion always got to me, and made my eyes fill with tears.

Afterwards, we almost always dined at La Brasserie, in Brompton Road. It is probably the most authentic brasserie in London. We went there because it stayed open until late, the food was reliably good, and we loved its lively atmosphere. The walls are painted or stained, possibly both, a nicotine colour. Over the years it has doubled in size, but lost none of its authenticity. The white linen table-cloths are protected by a paper one, so you can write on them – time for a quick game of noughts and crosses and a glass of champagne, while waiting for the first course. The waiters dress from neck to toe in black, with long white pinafores from the waist. Over the years we had seen many well- known personalities there, such as the singer Petula Clark and the cricketer – as he then was – Imran Khan.

As we had missed out on the Proms, we decided to make up for it, a little bit, by going there for dinner, after seeing the electrocardiologist.

6 September 2004

We went back to Spain. Always on the move, except that now we both needed to be. If we kept moving fast enough, perhaps the disease wouldn't catch up. We could out- manoeuvre it. But it would prove to be never far behind. In fact, I think it had already moved on ahead. It would lurk around a corner, waiting to inflict another blow, each time ever more deadly.

Our week in Spain was one of them. Alan had a bad fall when he tripped up a step.

We had parked in an underground car park in the centre of Marbella. We were off to have coffee and churros, basically a long thin doughnut, in our favourite little café. Alan loved churros. Leaving by the stairs, to the promenade above, he went down. He broke a piece off the end of his front tooth. There was blood everywhere, from where he hit his lip on the edge of the step. Fortunately, a Spanish couple came to our rescue, and called for an ambulance. We were taken to the local accident and emergency. The doctor saw Alan straight away, and he had to have two stitches, where the tooth had gone through his lip. They did it without anaesthetic, because that would have been the equivalent of one of the stitches. Alan was very brave. I sat beside him, and held his hand, but I couldn't watch because of my own needle phobia! That was the end of the coffee and churros – lunch too!

Needless to say he got an infection, that poor immune system again. This necessitated a visit to the GP, in the nearby town of San Pedro, for a prescription for an antibiotic cream. Eating was uncomfortable, and he looked as though he had been in a prize fight, so we didn't have the desire to go to some of our usual restaurants. This would turn out to be our last holiday in Spain on our own.

5 October 2004

The MND Association Regional Care Development Adviser came to visit. This was our first direct contact with the organisation. Unfortunately she was about to leave her job, with no immediate replacement. However, during her visit we were given various useful tips. We covered what to expect, and how we might wish to prepare for the effects of the disease in the future, a little as we had done with the neurologist.

Her visit also resulted in our being put in touch with an MND Association Visitor who would come to see us, mainly I think, to try to give us emotional support. We were given some information about organisations that might be able to help, but I never felt encouraged to make contact, as they were apparently overstretched.

Amongst the useful tips that we were given, one was to maintain, and even increase, Alan's calorie intake, via fortified drinks. Apparently, it had been found that MND sufferers need more calories. These drinks are prescribed, and are an easy way of topping up. Alan started to have them between meals, and we managed to maintain his weight, certainly until just over four months before he died. This was the last time we were able to weigh him at home. As it turned out, they also helped in the latter stages of the disease – before he had the feeding tube – because of the sheer effort of eating.

8 October 2004

Alan went to the Royal Brompton Hospital for his pacemaker. He would be there for three days, and I think it was at this point that we really began to feel the effect of the disease on our life, and our lack of ability to control what happened.

We decided to have lunch at La Brasserie, before we went to the hospital. It gave us something to look forward to, and take our minds off the operation. The restaurant was within walking distance, although I must admit, I tried to persuade Alan that we should take a taxi after lunch. Alan insisted on walking.

He had only recently agreed to use a stick. His left foot and toes had begun to drop. It was this which had caused him to trip on the step in Spain, and when we got back home he had finally agreed to use the walking stick. Until then he had been very reluctant. He didn't want to give in to the disease, and using the stick represented another level of deterioration. I was more concerned that he might break a bone. I also thought people would be less likely to shy away from helping a man with a stick. To me the humiliation and danger of falling, and not being able to get up was worse than giving in to the disease. Our views were different. Alan finally gave in to my requests, only because his falls became much more frequent.

On our way from the restaurant, he fell. A passer-by, on the other side of the road, saw the fall and rushed over to help me get him up. We arrived at the hospital with grazed pride, but otherwise only grazed knuckles.

The ever-increasing incidents of falling resulted in the physiotherapist recommending light-weight foot splints. They were made for both feet, as it would be only a matter of time before Alan would get 'foot drop' in both feet. The foot splints fitted inside the shoes, and helped to keep the foot and toes lifted which in turn reduced the propensity to trip, for a while.

The operation itself went well, but Alan developed a blood clot in his left arm, soon after. The pacemaker was inserted, naturally on his left side. He wasn't allowed to move the arm much, and it started to swell up. Guessing the cause, we went off to our GP. He thought it very unlikely a clot was the cause of the swelling, and thought it more likely to be a skin infection. He wanted to prescribe antibiotics. Knowing our ability to attract the unusual – after all Alan had MND – I suggested it might be a good idea to have Alan checked for a blood clot, and not wait to see if the antibiotics did the trick. The GP referred him to the local hospital, the same hospital where we saw Alan's neurologist. They kept him in for three days, to do tests. Alan didn't want to stay in hospital. He would have preferred to be allowed to go home and return for whenever they booked the tests. They wouldn't agree. It was easier to arrange the tests if he stayed in hospital, but Alan wasn't happy.

He did have a clot. It was caused by the enforced lack of movement of the arm, after the pacemaker operation. Why he wasn't prescribed heparin at that point, I don't know. Surely, it would have saved him getting a clot, and having to be in hospital again?

As soon as he was home from hospital, I took all his clothes, and put them straight into the washing machine, while he went upstairs to have a bath. He hadn't had a bath or a shower for three days. It didn't occur to me until after he came out, that he had been too nervous to do either alone, and he had not wanted to admit to it. The disease was hitting his confidence. I know he would have hated not being able to have a bath or shower – and no one bothered. He was fastidious about cleanliness, possibly as a result of his natural tendency to get infections. From then on, I would do everything I could to keep him out of hospital, or at least try to be with him.

He was prescribed heparin injections, to dissolve the clot. The alternative medication, in tablet form, wasn't appropriate, owing to the risk of bruising and haemorrhaging from one of his ever-increasing falls.

A further trip to Spain was abandoned, because Alan had to have the injections until early December. He was too nervous that something would go wrong while we were away, and I would have to deal with it on my own. For a while we still tried to go. In order to do so, I needed to try to overcome that needle phobia of mine, so I could give him the heparin. Due to the weakness in his hands, he didn't have the ability to give it to himself.

A very kind nurse in the hospital, showed me how to do it. First, I had to practise by pushing a needle into the peel of an orange. Apparently, it feels very similar to pushing a needle through human skin. Then I made my first attempt on Alan. My hand was shaking so much! I kept thinking Alan was braver than me, to be letting me do this. I didn't look at his face while approaching him with the needle. It was the first time in the illness that I really had to swallow hard, and just get on with it. There would be many more times. It is amazing what one can do when necessity dictates. I just wish it hadn't dictated.

Not using the left arm after the operation, caused the muscles to weaken even faster. It would prove impossible to reverse this. Furthermore, the deterioration in the right hand was becoming more apparent. It had started to affect Alan's writing, so for the next few months he practised writing paragraphs from the newspaper, to try to help. We had read in the MND Association's magazine "Thumb Print", how someone else had done this. It was worth a try.

Emotionally, we were feeling the effect of more and more losses, and so it was that Alan contacted Dignitas for the first time. He tried hard to live with the disease. In fact he tried to the end, but now was the time to prepare his exit plan; the exit plan this country would not give him.

9 November 2004

An architect came to the house to discuss converting the down-stairs cloakroom into a shower facility. We also wanted to alter the access to the house, to enable me to get Alan in and out in a wheelchair, should the need arise. I say we, but Alan didn't really want to think about either of these things. He had made his plans for when the disease became too much. But I kept thinking, what if it doesn't work out as he expects? What is intolerable? Only Alan would know when life was intolerable for him. In the meantime, I wanted to ensure I could look after him at home, and try to make sure I could cope.

Neither of us wanted him to have to go into a nursing home, es-pecially after our recent experience of hospitals. I couldn't believe they would be able to cope with Alan's illness any better than hospitals, and they had proved woefully inadequate at looking after him.

Making the alterations was a means to help me cope at home. But building has a habit of not going to plan, and brings with it additional stress. It didn't help that I knew how little Alan liked building work. Would it have been better not to have it done? But then I could not have looked after Alan at home, as I did right to the end. Was it worth it just for that? Was it worth all the screams of frustration, which I know made him feel more helpless? But what could I do? With all my feelings pent up, I think that would have made me ill as well!

The plumber was subjected to one of my fits of utter frustration. Just as the shower room was finally reaching completion, only weeks before we would need it, as it happened, we discovered that he had put the pipes wrongly. The only simple way to overcome it was to have the floorboards up – something I had tried to avoid all along –and redirect the pipes. Alan heard me use expletives that I had never used before. I would find many more opportunities from that moment on.

Had I really done the best for Alan, by making alterations he may not have wanted? Did I concentrate on things that weren't important? I don't think so, but I don't know. I do know it meant I was able to look after him at home to the end, and as things turned out, perhaps it was for the best. Nevertheless, it wouldn't stop me wondering for a while after he died whether I had done the right thing, because of the enormous physical and emotional energy that had been required to organise everything to look after him. It had a detrimental affect on me, and therefore on him. The only person who could really tell me whether it was worth it, isn't here now.

The losses would affect us differently. While we were beginning to grieve together, we were also grieving apart, because we were coming at the disease from a different viewpoint. As a result, it wasn't always possible to be in tune with the other's grief.

Taking a Chance

Mid December 2004

We finally managed a weekend away, just after Alan's seventieth birthday. He had decided against a big party in the end. He didn't feel up to one. He couldn't dance the night away, so he preferred the idea of two small celebrations: one with the family, the other would be a lunch with his golf friends at his club in London, in the first week of January.

Michael came from Australia for the family celebration, just as he had for his father's sixtieth birthday. Then it had been a surprise. We had booked Alan's favourite local restaurant. We knew the owners well, and they had ensured that we would have our usual large round table. But there was an extra place laid. We were looking at the extra chair, and about to say something to the owners, when Michael appeared from the kitchen. The tears welled up in Alan's eyes, and mine. It was the best birthday present he could have given his father. For Alan's seventieth, however, Michael gave us advance notice, but his presence was no less emotional. The lunch was a happy occasion, as we all made an effort to put aside our concerns and forget that Alan had the death sentence hanging over him.

There were a number of things that Alan was now finding much harder. We had cancelled the annual trip to St Moritz, which was a major blow to us both. It was obvious he wouldn't be able to ski, and even walking looked ambitious. It no longer seemed appropriate to pursue the holiday. For the moment though, life was still pretty good. It had been quite a year, but life was closer to "normal" than it had been for a few months. The need for Alan's exit plan looked some way off, but it helped him to know it was there.

Then one night I was watching a late news programme on television. One of the items covered a doctor in China who was conducting operations on patients with spinal cord injuries, or diseases such as MND. The report indicated that he was having some success. The procedure involved the use of olfactory ensheathing cells, cells taken from the nasal tissue of unborn foetuses. I can understand how some would abhor the idea, but we were desperate.

I quickly requested the transcript of the programme, and obtained a copy of the video from the production company that had filmed the item. We needed a miracle. Could this be it?

We found out that there was a long waiting list, so we didn't waste any time in sending an e-mail to the hospital in China, to find out if Alan could be accepted for the procedure. On Christmas Day morning we had our reply. He would be considered for the operation. It seemed like a gift from heaven. It made our Christmas, and gave us hope where before we had none.

26 December 2004

On Boxing Day, my mother, Alan and I went for a walk in the gardens where I work. Going for a walk on Boxing Day had become a tradition. We liked to walk off the excesses of Christmas Day and get some fresh air. But this year was different.

Alan insisted my mother and I go for a 'good' walk, on our own. We left him walking slowly along the path above the long canal. This way he could walk on the flat and avoid steps. But I didn't want to go far, because he had recently started to use two sticks. As my mother and I walked away, I watched him leaning over the two sticks, and walking forward so slowly. I was terrified he would fall, but had to let him do it. He needed to do it. I couldn't bear the thought of what the disease was doing to him. He seemed so vulnerable, and I felt so helpless to do anything to prevent it. Oh, how I hoped China would give us the miracle!

The next few weeks were largely spent in trying to get our slot on the waiting list, at the hospital in China. We had been accepted, but this was only the beginning. The hospital gave us details of others with MND who had gone through the procedure, so we could find out how they had got on. Most were from Holland, and the success seemed to vary according to what stage the disease had reached, prior to treatment. Alan was still managing to do most things. We felt that, if we could at least stabilise the symptoms, it was worth going. The sooner the better, and even if it didn't work, we felt as though we were doing something.

I suppose we could have gone on another cruise or just spent time together. But we had been very lucky. We had done so much. The disease wasn't lucky, of course. It was probably about as unlucky as one could get, other than finding oneself in a country where war had suddenly broken out, with no obvious means of escape. But perhaps we could escape.

So when we were offered a slot for the operation in June, we accepted. I believe that, had it not been for this little piece of hope, Alan would have gone to Switzerland to die, while he could still make the journey reasonably easily on his own. For him to go alone, would have necessitated him going before he was ready to die – before he found the disease intolerable. For him to be forced to do this, because of the law here, was something I found inhuman, but I would have supported him in whatever he chose to do. How could I watch him suffer? It was beyond my comprehension.

Trying to find ways to prolong Alan's quality of life was my only goal. But I could never get ahead of the disease. I came close on occasions. Whatever the disease threw at us, I could not give up – not until he gave up. I needed him to live at home for as long as he wanted to live, with the maximum of control over his life. I needed this for both of us. But sometimes I think he was cross with me for trying to stay ahead. It made him think about something he didn't want to think about. I wish I hadn't had to do it. I am still not sure whether I did the right thing. I wish I hadn't had to think about it at all. Why did he have to have a disease with nothing in the armoury to fight it, and little to ease the suffering? A disease without hope. But not to have fought would have meant giving up; giving up on him. I couldn't do this, not until he decided he had had enough.

But neither of us could know, with any accuracy, when he would no longer want to go on. Alan had some idea of what he could stand. I remember when the occupational therapist and physiotherapist came from the hospice to make suggestions for changes to the house. We had a discussion about whether to install a through-the-floor lift, which would take a wheelchair, or whether to install a stair lift. They said that once Alan's trunk went, referring I think to the large muscles which support the spine, he would no longer be able to use a stair lift. There wasn't any space for a through-the-floor lift, so eventually we went for the stair lift. Besides he had made up his mind, while they were talking and announced: 'The day my trunk goes, that'll be it. I'll be off to Dignitas.' He made his wishes very clear. In his view, when his trunk went, that was the point his life would not be worth living. But what would we need to cope with before that? I had no idea. I wanted to be sure we were prepared and we didn't know if the operation in China would work. It was a long shot.

The stairs had to be altered, to accommodate the stair lift. More building work! Knowing how much Alan hated the disruption building work always caused, before the disease let alone now, didn't make it easy. I was always asking myself: 'Should I be doing this?' But it was done. It was done either side of the New Year. And just before the screed went down, to level the floor where the stairs had been, Alan tripped. He fell through the plaster board of the hall wall. We were lucky; he was much shaken, but only grazed his shoulder. Nevertheless, it was a nasty wound. The wall was easily repaired, and fortunately Alan was as well, on this occasion. But from now on, I was terrified he would do something that would affect his mobility, increase the speed of the disease or result in a hospital stay. Worse still, would be an injury that would prevent us from going to China.

Mid February 2005

It was shortly before my birthday when I went down with flu. This was the last thing I needed. Since Alan was first diagnosed with MND, I tried to avoid being in contact with any illness, for fear he would catch it. We had our flu jabs, but this particular bug obviously got through the fire wall. Alan went down with it soon after me (no surprise there, with his immune system!). I wasn't able to take to my bed to recover, because Alan had started to need help with personal care even before he caught my flu.

Using his hands was already becoming limited. He couldn't shave himself properly. He had always used an electric shaver, but now it was rather heavy for him, and he needed help with anything fiddly. These were inconveniences. One might say they were minor inconveniences. But they were of enormous significance. It wasn't as though he would one day be able to do them again. Once he stopped being able to do something that would be it, forever.

In the middle of me being ill with the flu, Alan had another fall, and it made me realise how vulnerable we were. Caroline had phoned in the morning to check if there was anything we needed. She was going to the shops, and knew I wasn't well. She lived close by. I had managed to go out the day before, to do my weekly shop, so there wasn't anything, except a newspaper. She dropped the paper in. Later I started to get things out for lunch, and called Alan into the kitchen. But then he started calling me. I found him on the floor, in front of the sofa. He had tried to push up out of the sofa with his arms. As he had done so, it had moved back, and he had slipped down to the floor. I tried to help him to get up, but felt too weak, probably because of the flu. Previously he had been able to help me, but now he couldn't. I panicked.

Without realising it, we had edged forward and toppled over one of those plateaus. Until that moment, we had been able to cope with most of the effects of the disease by ourselves, including falls. Not being able to get Alan up by myself frightened the life out of me.

I called Caroline. It was a Saturday afternoon, and most of our neighbours were out. Besides I didn't like to bother them if there was another way, and I assumed his daughter wouldn't mind. I didn't know what else to do. I think I must have caught her at a bad moment. I can't remember what was said, but the tone of the response was indicative of this, and I wished I hadn't found it necessary to ask. Anyway, she came with her partner.

When they arrived I let them in and while they got Alan up, I started to put lunch on the table in the kitchen. I was on automatic pilot by this time. Sadly, they were not in a position to notice that both Alan and I were in shock. Much as it had been when strangers had come to our aid in the street, they checked that he was all right and that was it. They left.

Except that wasn't it. This was the first time that either of us had really felt the humiliation of the disease. It had pierced our armour.

What I did not know, and should have known, if someone had taken the trouble to tell me, was that we could have called the ambulance service for assistance. I only learnt this when I mentioned what had happened to the Macmillan Nurse who came to see us soon after. In fact it was recommended that we should call them in the future.

This incident was probably the first time that I was made to feel isolated. I wasn't sure which way to go for help, and it would become an all-too-frequent feeling. Alan was clearly aware that the disease was taking its toll on me, as well as on him. The flu and my emotional state were symptoms of this, and he was worried. He didn't want help for himself:

he wanted it for me. Of course, anyone who stops to think about it would realise that helping me to cope meant he was being helped. But he was worried about me, and the person he felt would be most likely to know how to help, and give me the support he wanted for me, was my mother. So he asked her to come to stay.

She dropped everything, packed a bag and came. However, if Alan thought my mother would arrive, send me to bed and make a fuss of me, he had got that bit wrong. That was not her style of nursing, not her style at all for that matter, at least not in my experience. She had always been good at rapidly assessing a situation and delegating, not unlike Alan. And that was what she did when she arrived. There was little more she could do; after all she was nearly eighty. But someone had to do, which in the circumstances left only me. This was fine for everyone, except the person Alan depended on; everyone, but the person Alan relied on to fight for his best interests. If there was one single period in our life, when we fought for each other more than at any other time, it was from this point onward. We had to, because we could only really depend on each other, and even then the disease did everything it could to get in the way.

My mother tried her best; she would do more to help us than anyone else during Alan's illness, without ever having to be asked. But preferring to delegate, she suggested I should get in touch with Alan's doctor. She did this as soon as she arrived because she could see that if I wasn't supported quickly, I wouldn't be in a fit state to look after Alan. She could also see that I wasn't in any state to think clearly for myself; so she did do that bit for me.

By now Alan had gone down with the flu. I think he had been sickening for it when he slid off the sofa. As if that wasn't enough, my mother went down with it as well. Nowhere near recuperated myself, I now had my mother, as well as Alan, to look after; so much for Alan's plan of getting help for me. And my mother has always been a lousy patient. I took her home as soon as I could. I didn't have the energy for another flu victim in the house.

The whole flu episode laid me especially low. I was on a huge downer and I think it was only the thought of China that pushed me on and gave me the energy to contact others for help. The flu had made me realise that no matter how much I wanted to do everything for Alan, I just couldn't.

I can't remember who I contacted first. I think it was the doctor, and as a result the district nurse came, then social services and the Macmillan Nurse. One of them attempted to get a Marie Curie nurse, to relieve me for a couple of nights, to help me recover, but they were unable to get one. The social services organised short–term carer support for Alan, and gave us the name of a local care company for us to organise help for ourselves.

Getting outside involvement was a really difficult, but necessary step for us. We had always been self-reliant, and wanted to remain that way. If I could have continued to look after Alan alone, I would have much preferred to do that. Many times I wanted to close the door on the world, because fighting all the time for help felt like a waste of energy, and it would be at the expense of our privacy. Achieving the right balance would be hard.

However, on this occasion something did happen, and it was enough for the moment. A carer started to come every morning, to help Alan with any aspects of his personal care that he could no longer manage. This gave me some respite, but more importantly, it was supposed to put our relationship back on its original footing.

Apparently the effect of having to act as a person's carer, when you have been their partner, has a detrimental effect on both individuals, and potentially on the relationship. Alan didn't want someone else doing things for him; not me, not anyone. He didn't want to have to rely on someone else for his needs. There wasn't an easy solution, but it was agreed that I needed help.

Having someone to help with Alan's personal care became essential, rather than merely enabling us to have a normal relationship. However, it was a wonderful ideal and worth striving for, which is why I could never understand why people insisted on referring to me as his main carer. I was his partner.

The disease, because of the disabilities it caused and pressures it brought, did have a negative impact on our relationship. Of necessity, the person with the disease becomes disproportionately more dependent on the other. This is likely to be humiliating in some way or another, no matter how hard one tries to make it otherwise. In Alan's case it was especially difficult to accept, because he had always been very much in control. For me the term carer added to the negative impact of the disease, not least because he had always been my protector, not the other way round. It was a role he didn't want to lose, and I didn't want him to lose it either. It gave him dignity and made me feel safe.

Every time I was referred to as Alan's 'carer' or 'main carer,' I flinched. What is more, it made it sound like a job. But I cared for him because I wanted to. I was doing it for love not money. To me the title was inappropriate. It may have described the reality of the situation, but it was not what Alan wanted for me. For my part, I didn't want him to feel any more dependent and helpless than the disease already made him. I wanted to remain his partner. As his partner I wanted to care for him, just as he still wanted to care for me. It was another reason for wanting China to fulfil our hopes.

3 March 2005

My birthday had been and gone in the midst of the episode with the flu, and now we had a progress appointment with the neurologist.

The appointment was also an opportunity to discuss China. He had heard about the procedure, but knew nothing of its potential to stabilise the disease. However, he understood our need to try, and was supportive of our decision to go. He said that he looked forward to hearing all about it on our return.

With the flu behind us, and China on the horizon, we felt positive once more. We treated ourselves to a day out in nearby Windsor. We were also looking forward to the imminent return of Alan's son and his family to the UK.

I drove to Windsor, because Alan wasn't confident about driving the car. That day when we couldn't get him up from the floor by ourselves, had left him wondering if his arms were strong enough to control the steering wheel. We decided that we would find a safe place on the way back, so he could have a go at driving, just to see if he had enough strength. Unfortunately, after a very short distance, he had to pull over. His fears realised; something else taken away. We hoped he would be able to drive again after China. We both needed to be hopeful for the other. Whatever doubts we had then, we didn't want to show it. We had to remain positive. But he never drove a car again.

21 March 2005

The stair lift was installed. Initially Alan wouldn't use it. It meant giving up something else to the disease. He persevered, hauling himself up the stairs using the handrail. However, the lift was used to send my cup of tea upstairs each morning. He followed. At the top of the stairs he took the cup from the lift, and brought it in to me. He knew how much I loved my cup of tea in bed. Alan used to wake up much earlier than me, and I remember how he used to come back to bed with me. He liked a biscuit with his tea. He let me slowly come round, amused at how anyone could drink their tea while still remaining under the bed covers. Once I surfaced we would chat and sometimes more. He would bring me a cup of tea for as long as he could. He was determined.

He did give in to a battery-operated bath lift. For sometime now he had only been able to shower, which he did by sitting on a bath seat across the bath. He couldn't get himself up out of the bath safely. But he enjoyed a relaxing bath, so the bath lift provided a solution, for a while at least.

Added to everything else, Alan found it increasingly difficult to feed himself. Using a knife and fork had become virtually impossible. We went through a range of cutlery, trying to find something suitable. The help of the hospice was enlisted in our search and they suggested a mobile arm support.

This device, which would enable Alan to maintain control and therefore dignity, in at least one area of his life, was one of the few things in the whole of the illness to be readily offered. It was organised through the Oxford Centre for Enablement*. It was marvellous. It had a bracket that could be fitted onto a table or wheelchair. Alan rested his arm in a support, which was designed so that it could swing on the bracket, and direct the spoon (secured to his hand by a band) into his mouth. With the exception of the environmental control system, which came later, this piece of equipment probably did most to lift his spirits. We had been forced to deal with so many losses, and his not being able to feed him-self, would soon have been another, had it not been for this piece of equipment.

It meant Alan could choose how he ate his food, and how long he took over it. There were some flavours he liked to mix, and some he liked to keep separate, and although I tried when I fed him, I didn't al-ways get it right. He would say 'No, no, no.' It was said jokingly, but he was frustrated that he had to go through this. Sometimes, when I was feeding him, my attention would be diverted. He would be left staring at the spoon, hovering in mid-air, with his food on it. 'Excuse me,' he would say, in a tone that was meant to remind me of what I was sup-posed to be doing. We could and did laugh at the time, but it was frus-trating for him. It was humiliating, and I chastised myself whenever I did it. For the moment, this piece of equipment gave him back that all-important control and self-respect. And it helped me; not just because I didn't have to feed him, but because I knew what it meant to him.

The same piece of equipment helped some months later, when Alan lost the ability to write. By adapting it, it was possible for him to sign his name. You could still distinguish it as his signature, and with it he was able to sign my Christmas card. This was little more than four months before he died. My Christmas card was the last thing he signed.

24 March 2005

Alan saw a speech therapist for the first time. The neurologist re-ferred Alan, via the GP, having discussed it with us at the last progress appointment. At this moment, there was no detectable effect on his speech, but it enabled the speech therapist to monitor any deterioration, and advise him on ways to save his voice.

She suggested he use short phrases, or a simple 'yes' or 'no' when this would suffice, and try not to talk for long at any one time. It was very important that he should not put a strain on his voice in any way, for example by shouting. He should limit his use of the telephone, which apparently also puts more strain on the voice than talking face to face.

Early April 2005

Apart from the day-to-day, everything was now geared to organ-ising the trip to China, and keeping us both able to undertake the trip. We did all we believed that could minimise Alan's deterioration, includ-ing diet, physiotherapy and massage.

On top of the deterioration in the strength of his hands, his fingers were tending to curl over, and it was becoming harder for him to straighten them. To help him, the physiotherapist arranged for left and right hand splints to be made. These were designed to keep the hands and fingers straight. Alan wore them for about half an hour twice a day, and sometimes for longer periods. He could wear them while he watched television. It was suggested he wear them overnight, but he found this too uncomfortable, and was also worried that he might inadvertently knock me out!

We tried to live life as normally as possible, but whenever we relaxed the disease found a way to remind us of its presence. One night, I was going up to bed, and the next moment I heard a crash. I had heard this noise enough times now to know it meant only one thing. Alan had fallen. I had left him to make his own way up. He had started to use the stair lift, having finally given in to it. He had also started to use a walker to get around inside, as well as outside, the house.

I ran downstairs. I don't know exactly how he fell, but he had managed to fall backwards with the walker on top of him. This time it was a bad fall. From where he landed, I could tell he had banged his head on the edge of the door frame. I could see the damage to the frame, but in order to see what Alan had done to his head, I needed to get down on the floor behind him, and raise it. There was a huge gash. I remember saying: 'Sorry darling, but this time we have to go to hospital.' I don't remember him saying anything, not until we were in the hospital. I went on automatic pilot again.

He had fallen near the phone and the cupboard under the stairs, where I keep old clean towels, so that I was able to grab a towel and press it against the gash in his head, while with the other hand I dialled 999. As instructed, I left him for a second, to open the front door for the ambulance staff; so they could come straight in as soon as they arrived. They arrived shortly afterwards, to find us on the floor together, with me dressed only in my T-shirt and underpants. I was still holding Alan's head, and pressing a towel against it, to stem the blood. His head needed stitches. I got dressed, while Alan was taken to the ambulance. They asked if I felt all right to drive. I said I was; as ever putting on an outward appearance of being able to cope. I followed in the car, so I could bring us both back later. We spent most of the night at the hospital, in Accident and Emergency, waiting for someone to become free to remove the bits of door-frame from Alan's injury, and clean and repair the wound. It was a long deep cut, requiring quite a few stitches, but at least there seemed to be no other damage and we could return home together.

From then on, Alan started to wear an ice hockey helmet to protect his head against any similar injuries from further falls. It was his idea, and his daughter got one for him. Of course, this did not protect the rest of his body, but it made him feel more confident. As his ankles weakened, so they began to turn over when he walked. The foot supports he wore in his shoes helped with this problem, as did elastic ankle supports. He also wore elastic supports for his weakening wrists, so he could use the walker. He balanced himself over it and used his weight to move it forward. He was determined to continue walking and remain independently mobile.

In order for me to have some peace of mind when I had to leave Alan alone in the house, I managed to persuade him that we needed to install a Helpline. Local councils organise these Helplines, but in our case it was paid for by the MND Association. It would be one of the few things we didn't have to pay for ourselves. I was encouraged to accept this benefit because any assistance would help our funds to stretch further, and I didn't know how long we had.

The Helpline meant that, for now at least, Alan didn't have to have someone with him all the time. He didn't want someone there all the time. We all need space. The system raised help when needed. By pressing a button on a wrist-band (there were other methods for activating the alarm, but this one was best for Alan), it automatically dialled through to an operator at another location. The operator would ask what help was needed and act accordingly. It proved valuable reassurance for us both. He could be independent, but help was at hand if he fell in the house, or another emergency arose when he was on his own.

11 April 2005

Alan was determined that we should still try and have some time away at the apartment in Spain, and besides he felt it would do us both good before we went to China. Michael agreed to come with us to help, which made it possible for me to relax and have a much-needed holiday.

Between us we managed to persuade Alan to use a wheelchair, which we hired in Spain. He wasn't happy about using one, but I didn't want any accidents before China. It also allowed us to do more. Alan could only walk short distances now, and only then with the walker. Negotiating the steps to and from the apartment would have been impossible without Michael.

The weather was absolutely perfect: not too hot. It was ideal for sitting out on the terrace with Alan and reading. Michael made full use of the swimming pool, while Alan and I lazed on the terrace. We both relaxed, and it was lovely to have time to read or lie out in the sun, doing nothing. I remember thinking of some of our holidays before the shadow of MND crossed our lives.

There was that first holiday abroad, in 1982. We ended up going to Morocco. It was a last-minute booking. We stayed in an apartment in Agadir and while there, we booked a day trip to Marrakesh. Alan liked Marrakesh, but I wasn't so keen. The pestering to buy in the souk made me uneasy, and I couldn't wait to get out. Alan had never seen me move so fast past shops! The children running after us, laughing and shouting 'Fish and chips,' the only English they knew, did make me laugh. But it was the poverty, and seeing children begging in the streets, which upset me. I hadn't encountered it before, at close range.

Also I had to use a dreadful toilet in Marrakesh. It was outside the café that the tour company took us to, close to the dusty street. I had to go down some steep steps. There was a boy outside. He tore off a piece of toilet paper, from a roll, and handed it to me in exchange for money. I went into the toilet – it was a hole in the ground. There wasn't a lock on the door, so I had to hold it shut with my hand while I crouched down, and with no form of lighting, I endured the disgusting stench in utter blackness. When I came out there was nowhere to wash my hands. The boy put out his hand for me to shake and smiled. I couldn't help wondering what germs passed between us, and related the experience to Alan, when I returned to the cafe. He thought it was very funny. I suppose it was, and he was more able to take these things in his stride, perhaps because of his RAF days in Egypt.

But we enjoyed Morocco so much, that we went back the following year. We learnt from our experience though. Rather than join a tour, we hired a car to go to Taroudant, a lovely, old walled town. We stopped to eat where we wanted, selecting hotels that were likely to have decent toilets. On the way to Taroudant, we stopped to take photographs in the desert. We thought we were in the middle of nowhere, but suddenly we were surrounded by children, clamouring to have their photos taken. Of course they wanted money too, but even now I can still remember their shouts of delight and picture their happy faces.

Then there was the safari holiday in Kenya. Ever since my parents let me stay up late to watch the Survival programme on television, I had dreamed of going to Kenya. We arrived in Mombassa to an official welcoming party! In fact it was for President Moi. As a result, for the first part of our journey to the game lodge, the roadside was lined with hundreds of people. There was music playing and the women were dressed in colourful African dress. The safari was everything I had hoped it would be, but it could not compare with the one we did in South Africa, a few years later. That time, we were taken out in open-top vehicles, and had our own tracker and driver. We were able to get really close to see the animals.

On one occasion, we found ourselves in the middle of a large herd of buffalo. They were almost close enough to touch, although we would have been foolhardy to have tried. They are one of the 'big five' and as such, very dangerous. As long as you stay sitting in the vehicle, they are unlikely to harm you.

On another occasion, we sat and watched as a mother giraffe stood by her baby, the two of them encircled by a group of hyenas, seeing a potential meal. The giraffe is not well designed for giving birth, and the baby had broken one of its legs in the process. The mother giraffe was trying very hard to push her baby into a standing position, but she couldn't do it. It was heartbreaking. No matter how hard she nuzzled and pushed, the baby was unable to stand, but she wouldn't leave it until she knew it was dead. She wouldn't desert the baby and leave it to the hyenas before then.

We had enjoyed some wonderful holidays, but probably the best holiday of all was the cruise in South America. The cruise ship was small enough to navigate large stretches of the Amazon River. At times the banks on either side were so close you felt you would be able to touch the vegetation, just like the buffalo when we were on safari. The inhabitants along the river banks came to greet us in their canoes. Some of the little vessels contained very young children, rowing on their own. No health and safety rules!

The final destination of the cruise was Buenos Aires. We didn't have to go far in this city to see couples dancing the tango. From the artists' quarter of La Boca, with its brightly painted little houses, to the bustling Sunday market at San Telmo, with its open- air-restaurants and live bands, the tango is the soul of this vibrant and beautiful city. And we had one particularly memorable experience: we had read that there were around thirty thousand taxi drivers in Buenos Aires. Somehow, we managed to get the same one two days running. He couldn't believe it any more than we could. We were waiting our turn in a queue, so it was completely by chance.

It was lovely lying in the sunshine in Spain, being able to look back at these holidays. We had been so lucky. It made me feel content and happy for the first time in ages. If only it could have lasted.

This trip made up for the September trip, which had been spoilt for both of us when Alan had his first bad fall, breaking a tooth and needing stitches in his lip. We ate out every evening and also managed to get some amusement from the wheelchair. Walking around the old town in Marbella, admiring the buildings, none of us noticed the un-covered drain ahead. Next thing we knew, there was a shout from Alan, as the front wheels descended down the hole. Fortunately, the wheels jammed in the hole before he fell out of the wheelchair, but it created a lovely picture in our minds, of the moment we nearly lost him down a drain! The three of us laughed. It was good to laugh and feel light-hearted. It seemed like ages since we had been able to be like this.

Alan was right: our week in Spain was just what I needed and seeing me happy, relaxed and smiling, made him happy. It had the de-sired effect – it did us both good.

19 April 2005

We arrived home fully refreshed. It was time to get everything ready for what would truly be the journey of a lifetime: our expedition to China.

Our Childhood - Seperated by the Years

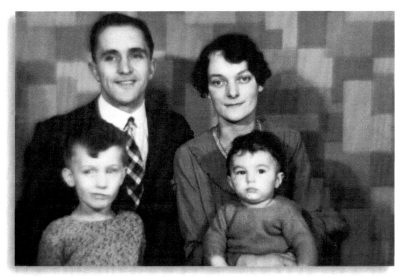

A family portrait

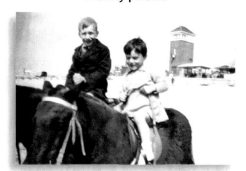

Holidays at Littlehampton

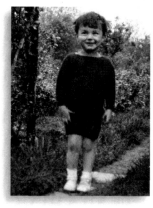

Up the garden path

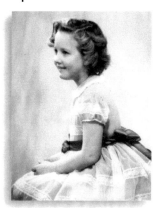

My favourite party dress

Making Our Way in the World before we Met

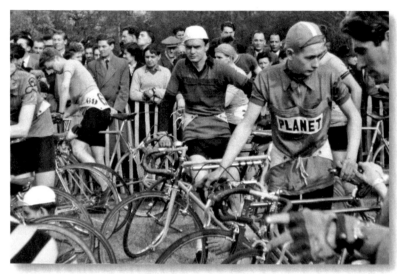

Preparing for the race

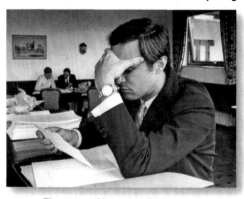

The young Managing Director

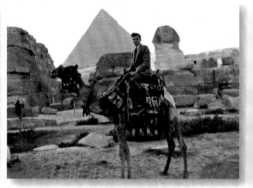

At the pyramids

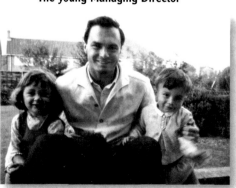

The proud father

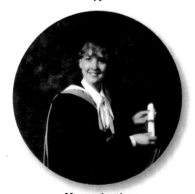

My graduation

Our Wonderful Life Together

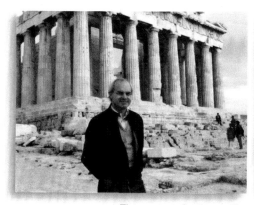 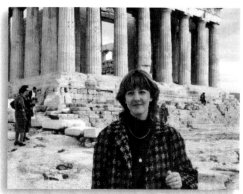

Time out at the Acropolis - a winter weekend in Athens

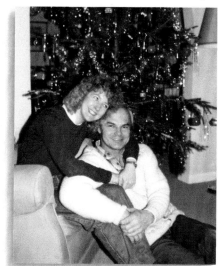 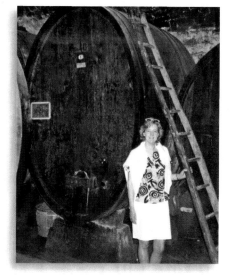

First Christmas   My fortieth in Tuscany

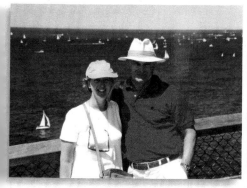 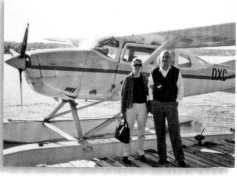

Together in Sydney   New Zealand and a flight over the volcanoes

Unaware that a Shadow was Falling

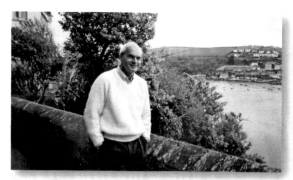

Fowey - Alan and his favourite jumper

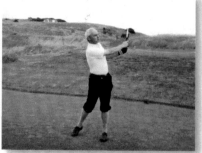

Alan loved his golf

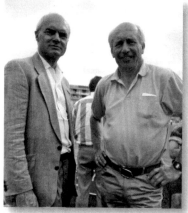

Two brothers at the cricket
for the last time

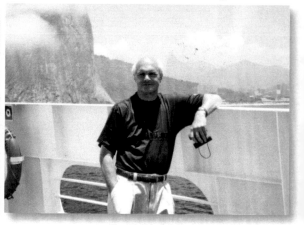

South America

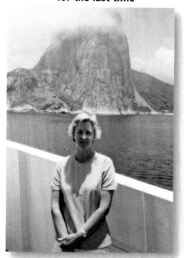

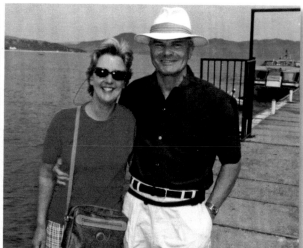

South America - our last carefree voyage

The Trip to China

Wednesday, 1 June 2005

This was it; the most important journey of our lives. I was filled with trepidation, but the fact that Michael was going to come with us for the first week, helped us to carry it out. His support meant a lot to us both.

We left for China, as though we were going on a long expedition. We had so much support luggage; everything we could think of which might be useful. There was a wheelchair that folded flat to allow it to be stowed in the hold. This was courtesy of Wheelchair Services. There was Alan's walker, courtesy of the hospice, also able to fold flat, that came with us into the cabin. There was the bath seat, Alan's foot/ankle splints, his energy drinks and the crash (ice hockey) helmet. Last, but by no means least, we took with us the 'piss pot', as I came to call it. There were few things to laugh about during the latter part of the illness, and we had been used to laughing a lot, so any opportunity to have some fun was utilised to the full, and giving this particular receptacle this derogatory name, gave me a perverse form of pleasure. It was naughty. But on some occasions I used this name because I was desperate, needing the pot quickly, for Alan. It was only the tone of my voice, and the expression in my eyes, which told someone whether I was using it in fun, or sheer frustration. But, whenever I said it, it was always to express an urgent need.

We didn't know what to expect, with regard to the facilities at the hospital, and so we took whatever might be essential for our survival. Probably the only thing missing was the kitchen sink. We understood that we might be in China for six weeks. Thankfully it turned out to be a lot less - less than three weeks. We learnt when we got there, that the hospital had refined the procedure. They had been able to do this via more reliable sources of olfactory ensheathing cells.

The flight out was not uneventful, and not because of Alan for a change! We were on an overnight flight to Beijing. In the middle of the night, he woke up because he wanted to go to the toilet. Well, in a way, I suppose it was because of Alan. The piss pot was in the luggage in the hold. We hadn't planned on using it on the plane. It was a stupid lack of forethought on my part, but I didn't know how I would be able to use it.

I had to wake Michael up from a deep slumber, so he could help me. He got his father up from the seat, and together we put the manual-handling belt round his hips. I had to use a manual-handling belt in situations where Alan's balance might be affected, situations in which he might otherwise have used his arms to steady himself – except that his arms weren't strong enough to do this any more. The belt went round him, so that it rested on his hips. The three of us then formed a procession to the toilet. His son was at the front, walking backwards to steady the walker. Alan propelled himself forward on the walker, while I steadied him from behind, with the belt. It must have looked as though we were trying to start a conga! Once there, Michael had to hold on to his father, as the walker wouldn't go over the toilet. I looked after that outside.

Luckily, the door to the toilet wouldn't shut, with both of them in there. Suddenly, Michael's face turned pale and his eyes glazed over. I saw it all happening in the mirror!

He had passed out, but somehow he was still standing and holding Alan. I grabbed Michael, and called one of the flight attendants sitting nearby. She took him. In the process, I moved in to hold on to Alan. Then the flight attendant helped me to get Alan back to his seat, leaving Michael recovering at the front of the plane. I adopted the role he had taken on the way to the toilet, proceeding in reverse, and guiding the walker from the front. Thankfully, Alan didn't need to go again until we got to China.

It would have been tremendously helpful if someone had taken the trouble to talk to us about some of the difficulties we would come up against with Alan's decreasing mobility. That way we could have been better prepared. When I was relating the story to either the district nurse or the Macmillan Nurse a few weeks later, because I had been wondering why something hadn't been invented for the problem we had encountered on the plane, one of them told me it had. There are bags that can be worn, which connect to a sort of condom via a tube*. If Alan had been wearing this on the plane, he could have had a pee without all the hassle and trauma. Later, once we knew about the device, it would come in handy both at home and when we went out.

Thursday, 2 June 2005

We arrived in Beijing, and were relieved that the airport staff turned out to be so helpful. A very modern small wheelchair was used to take Alan from his seat on the plane to the terminal building. I hadn't seen one before, and I haven't seen one since. It was small enough to go down the aisle of the plane. Our unusual baggage cleared customs without a hitch, and the three of us walked out onto the concourse. It was a massive space, somewhat intimidating, particularly in our circumstances.

We were expecting to be met at the airport by a member of staff from the hospital. We had been given a name, but she wasn't there when we arrived. I thought, 'God surely this isn't a scam, and we are going to have to turn round and go home!' I found a member of the airport staff to phone the hospital for us. The mobile telephone we had bought especially for the trip, supposed to work in China, wouldn't work. I was just beginning to really panic, when the person from the hospital turned up.

We had to spend the first two nights in a hotel. We knew this might happen if the room at the hospital wasn't ready. It sometimes occurs when the previous patient's departure is delayed. It was not ideal for all sorts of reasons, but the biggest problem was the height of the hotel bed: it was very low. Thank goodness Michael was with us. I wouldn't have been able to get Alan up from the bed on my own; something else I was not prepared for. I should have thought about it. The bed at home had not long been put up on blocks, so Alan could stand up from it without help. But what could I have done about it? It was probably just as well I didn't think of everything. We might never have gone!

On the plus side, the shower was separate from the bath. Access to it wasn't ideal, but it was manageable. It was easier than using the bath seat over the bath. Alan worked out an ingenious way of keeping the walker dry with his plastic mac, so he could use it to support himself under the shower. Increasingly, he was thinking of ways to help me to help him, now that his abilities had diminished considerably. Furthermore, he relied on the walker completely now, for getting around, so he wanted to protect it.

The two days in the hotel were an opportunity to see some of the tourist sites. We took a taxi round Beijing, and to Tian'anmen Square, which in 1989 became the venue for a demonstration that would leave many protestors dead, after the military went in to bring it to an end. I had seen Tian'anmen Square on television, but never appreciated the enormity of it. At one end is the Forbidden City, behind the Tian'anmen Gate. There was a large portrait of Chairman Mao, hanging on the wall of the Gate. The Great Hall of the People is on one side of the Square, and museums take up the length of the opposite side, while in the middle there stands a thirty metre high obelisk, commemorating the victims of the revolutionary struggle.

The taxi driver took us to the old part of Beijing, which is around the outside of the Forbidden City. It is a fascinating area with lots of little single storey shops, houses and restaurants nestled together.

On the way back to the hotel we drove past the site on which the

National Stadium for the 2008 Olympic Games was being built, the stadium which would become known as the Bird's Nest. We still had some way to go, as our hotel was on the outskirts of Beijing. We were all quiet by this time, wrapped up in our own thoughts. It had been a long day, especially as we were already tired out from the inevitable last minute preparations in the days leading up to the trip, and then the travelling.

Alan probably wondered whether he would see the Beijing Olympics as we drove past. In fact, he possibly wondered if he might be around for the ones in London, in 2012, if the operation was successful. It would have been only natural; he loved sport so much, and of course, there had been that first visit to the Olympics in London with Lionel, his brother, when he was still in his teens.

For me, seeing the stadium triggered a long string of memories associated with two people we knew who lived in Athens: a couple called George and Fifi.

Our friendship with George and Fifi was a thread that ran through much of our life. We had been to see them in November 2002, almost exactly a year before Alan was initially diagnosed as having MND. We thought it would be interesting to see what changes the Olympics were making to Athens, and at the same time, affording an excuse to catch up with old friends. Although we had kept in touch, we hadn't seen them in almost ten years; not since Alan retired.

They had been clients of his, but the relationship soon developed into more than just a business acquaintance. Alan attended their daughter's wedding with his own daughter.

It had all started because they owned a company that made and sold toys. They had invited Alan to go to Athens to discuss how he could help them. Ever the perfectionist, he prepared a professional presentation to promote his own company's expertise. He may have gone to more trouble than they expected. He ended up giving the presentation in their garden, and felt a little out of place, with his flip chart and other visual aids. But it was a beautiful sunny day, and one he would remember for the rest of his life. About halfway through, everyone got up and left him. He thought he had made some sort of faux pas until they began to return, one by one, with plates and plates of food. They had been so impressed by the trouble he had taken they were embarrassed. They wanted to make up for not being more welcoming. Over the years, they would more than make up for that occasion with their friendship.

One summer, they allowed us to use their boat, a small cruiser. We were looked after by the ship's captain and mate, who sailed us round lots of beautiful little Greek islands in the Ionian Sea. The weather was fantastic, except for the day when we had to ride out a hurricane! It could have been very scary. Everything went completely dark, and we could see the trees on the nearby island, pushed sideways by the force of the storm winds. Our captain had decided it would be better to sail out to sea for the duration of the storm, rather than remain anchored in the harbour. Although tossed about by some angry waves, we felt safe in his experienced hands – safe enough to watch the hurricane from the deck of the boat. Only when it was all over, did we venture back into the harbour, where we met a great deal of frantic activity. Divers were busily untangling the anchors of the boats there. That night we had an unexpectedly romantic dinner in a small taverna on the edge of the harbour. The only light was provided by candles, because the storm had cut off the electricity.

We spent quite a long time at the island of Kefalonia, moored in the delightful small harbour of Fiscardo. The captain organised a car to take us to the island's spectacular caves and a boat to go on Lake Melissani, an incredible semi-underground lake of clear turquoise and indigo water. On another day we sailed round to a long pale golden sandy beach. It was beautifully quiet with nobody else there – our own private beach for the afternoon.

If I had to pick one single highlight of that wonderful time, it would be sailing through the narrow waters of the Corinth Canal. Staring up at the steep rock face that enclosed us on either side, we had to crane our necks to see the top. A bridge, which spanned the canal, looked tiny from where we were on the boat. The blue of the sky, like the waters below us, reflected off the bright sand-coloured rock. It was just a short stretch from these waters to Athens, where George and Fifi met us, at the end of a perfect time together for me and Alan.

Whenever I thought of them, it always got me thinking of a meeting between Alan and George, in Geneva. George and Fifi rarely came to London, as they didn't like to leave their dog for long. Usually they chose to meet in Paris, but they were visiting friends in Geneva and asked Alan to fly over. I often went with him or joined him later, after his meetings, sometimes flying to Athens for a weekend, but not on this occasion. Alan was booked into a swish hotel, the Hôtel du Rhône, and given a large comfortable suite. An impressive bowl of fruit and a beautiful flower arrangement rested on one of the tables in the room. Alan thought, 'George must have some influence, for the hotel to have gone to so much trouble.' He picked the envelope out of the middle of the fruit, took the card from inside and started to read, *'Mr Woody Allen, Welcome to Genève ... (the) Director Wishes you a most enjoyable stay.'*

Alan couldn't wait to show me the card when he got home. While he was telling me the story, he was laughing at the thought of Woody Allen being taken to the room they would have given him, had they not made a mistake over his identity.

Another time, they lent us their apartment in Paris. It was close to the Boulevard St Germain, on the left bank, so we could have our breakfasts at the nearby café, Deux Magots. Before lunch, on one of the days, we sat and watched the world go by, whilst we sipped champagne at Fouquets, on the Champs Élysées. That was near a club Alan had taken me to, by accident, on our first ever trip to Paris. We often joked about it. He had wanted to take me to a show at the Moulin Rouge or the Crazy Horse, but they were both fully booked, so the hotel recommended another nightclub. It turned out to be a high-class strip club! There was a magician for one of the acts, and we did get a bottle of champagne, but there any similarities with the Moulin Rouge or the Crazy Horse ended.

These times had become so deeply and fondly etched in my memory. They were my life, our life. Yet they had felt like someone else's in that moment when the taxi pulled up at the hotel. But they weren't. We had been so lucky. Surely that luck wouldn't stop now.

Saturday, 4 June 2005

We were transferred to the Neurological Disorder Research and Treatment Centre of the Beijing Xishan Hospital. A car was sent by the hospital to fetch us.

I am not sure how I would have coped, for this first part of our stay, had Alan's son not come with us. Michael could be like his father in many ways: he was kind, considerate and would get on and help, without being asked or making a fuss. I would have to do most of our stay in China on my own, but his being there at the beginning allowed me to adjust.

After a while, we settled into a routine. With Alan's gentle reassurance and appreciation, I was able to manage alone, when his son left to go home. I didn't have any choice. I think I was the only person there without additional support for the duration of the stay. Alan did his best to make it as easy as possible, but there was only so much he could do. It wasn't easy. It was probably a little crazy of me to have attempted any of it, but I would have done anything to slow or cure the disease. Clearly

129

Alan was prepared to do the same. Having the controversial operation took great courage.

The hospital was located at the foot of the West Hills, approximately twenty-five kilometres outside the centre of Beijing. It focuses on research into neuro-repair, nerve regeneration and neurological functional recovery. Alan was one of their guinea pigs, and we had been made aware from the beginning, that the operation was very experimental, and clinical results varied from patient to patient. However, we were prepared to try. There was nothing else.

We arrived at the hospital, which looked a little neglected and tatty from the outside. We wheeled Alan through the dark, dingy corridors into an equally dark, dingy lift operated by a member of the hospital staff: a small lady, dressed in a rather tired-looking uniform. We were taken to the floor of the hospital that housed the wing designated for private, foreign patients run by Professor Hongyun Huang.

It all felt very strange, and only then did it dawn on me just exactly how scared I was. Everything seemed even more foreign and different than I had expected, and so much depended on our stay there. From the reception we were taken to our ward. This was to be Alan's and my bedroom and living quarters. Michael stayed in separate basic quarters close by. Though better than the areas we had passed through, our hospital wing and ward did not seem at all inviting.

As soon as the three of us were alone in the room, I burst into tears. I was thinking, 'What on earth have we done?' Seeing me cry, Alan also started to cry. I put my arms around him, but he told me to put my head in his lap. With enormous effort, he raised his hand over my head, and gently stroked it, trying to give me comfort. We cried together, not knowing what was going to happen. We felt very lost.

The room had two beds, and at one end there were two sinks, positioned under a large window. We had our own shower room and toilet. They were in a separate room, off to the right of the sink area. There was a chair, a telephone, a water-filtering machine and a television. There was nothing wrong with it; it was just that we were suddenly aware of the reality of our undertaking. In fact, once we became used to it, the room became our womb. In some ways it was better-equipped, and certainly better-staffed, than the NHS wards we would have to go to later, back at home. The nursing staff and doctors were very kind and always cheerful.

One of my first tasks was to register with the British Consulate in Beijing, just in case anything went wrong and we needed assistance. I had brought with me all the information that I might need, on the suggestion of one of the people I worked with at the gardening charity. She had also given me the details of another of the volunteers, whose husband had previously worked at the Consulate in Beijing. It was she who had kindly provided the necessary contacts, to make it as easy as possible for us when we got to China.

Soon after we arrived, the three of us went on an excursion to the local supermarket. We needed to buy cleaning products and equipment, as well as comfort provisions, including chocolate and a very good Chinese wine, to consume with our meals in the evening. The meals provided weren't bad, with a good choice of western and Chinese food, and we could and did send out for pizzas, for variety.

In order to take my mind off the reason we were at the hospital, I found occupational therapy in cleaning our room. The hospital staff washed the floors, but any other cleaning is left to the family of the patient, hence the need for cleaning items on our shopping list.

We discovered the internet room. This, together with the phone in our room, provided the link with those back home, and their e-mails helped to keep our spirits up. Furthermore, after the operation, we were able to keep them up-to-date with progress, and reading e-mails and sending replies helped to fill the time. The occasional phone call from my own family was an added bonus. Somehow, a voice at the other end of a line helps to make one feel much less alone, in a strange environment.

The laundry room provided me with further occupational therapy. This long narrow room had a large window, at the opposite end to the doorway. Washing machines and driers lined the wall to left of the doorway. There was a long sink for hand-washing, running the whole length of the wall, on the opposite side. Apart from enabling us to do our washing, while we were staying at the hospital, the laundry room acted as a meeting place for the family and friends of those who had accompanied the patients. We all had one very special thing in common. We were all on a quest for a miracle, and the laundry room provided a forum for an informal support group. Here we swapped information and tips for surviving the stay; for instance, how to get more towels or equipment such as shower chairs. This room was always busy, and there was great competition for the washing machines and driers. The machines would make an alarm noise when they had finished a load. Our room was close enough to hear the noise, and it gave Alan endless hours of amusement, because I would sit on the edge of my bed waiting for the alarm. As soon as I heard it, I shot out with our load, before anyone else could claim the machine. The high-pitched alarm of the machine mingles with the smell of soap powder, clean washing and friendly chatter in my memory of that laundry room.

The patients were from all over the world. This was the first time that Alan and I had come into contact with other people with MND. All were at a more advanced stage. The patient who occupied the room next to ours wasn't able to speak. I would hear him moaning and crying with frustration, because he couldn't make himself understood.

The fear that Alan would not be able to speak, and not be able to easily tell people what he wanted or felt, was bad enough, but now it was made a reality for me. It was to affect me deeply. From that moment on, I would never be able to get the sound of the sobbing out of my head. And when the time came that Alan too cried, because he also felt so helpless, I could hear that man – that poor man in the room next to ours in China. I didn't talk about it, not even to Alan, so how could he know the effect his crying had on me? But not long before he died I shouted 'Stop that!' at him. I was angry at the disease; for what it had done to him. I wanted Alan back as he was before the disease had invaded every part of him. I couldn't bear it. But Alan was so stunned that he stopped. It left me feeling guilty.

Sunday, 5 June 2005

The doctors didn't waste any time. They conducted pre-op tests including X-ray, ECG, EMG, lung function and blood tests. We had taken with us Alan's brain scan from 2004. Because of the pacemaker, he could no longer have an MRI scan. They took a video of Alan doing various activities. This was to establish a baseline, to try to determine what effect the operation had. The aim of the procedure for Alan's form of MND, was to stabilise and ideally improve, his neurological function; to at least prevent any further deterioration in what he was able to do.

For the video, Alan had to write on a piece of paper, and try to use a knife and fork. He also had to do exercises, to show the mobility and strength in his fingers, hands, arms and legs. He had to complete a questionnaire of his abilities, which was similar to the one which he had done for King's College. The doctors would compare all of this against what he could do at the end of our stay.

They briefed us on the procedure, and advised us that they expected to do it immediately after the weekend. This was good news. The sooner it was done, the sooner we would be able to go home. They told Alan that the procedure would be done under local anaesthetic. He needed to be awake, because they would have to drill two small holes through his skull (either side of the mid-point of the upper part of his forehead) to the frontal lobe of the brain. The olfactory ensheathing cells would then be injected into this area. The risks involved were similar to a lot of operations, and ranged from infection to haemorrhage and cardiac arrest. None of the risks seemed worse than the eventual effect of the disease.

I was particularly concerned that the doctors explain fully the details of the procedure to Alan. I had been told by one of the other relatives, while we were chatting in the laundry room, that her father had been quite traumatised by the experience. He hadn't appreciated what would happen. We did. Alan and I had read about it, but now I started to worry. I kept on asking the doctors, 'He won't be able to see the drill going in?' It didn't occur to me to ask if Alan would feel it. Alan didn't ask either. Even now I don't know if he did feel anything; we were so intent on getting our miracle. The doctors told us he wouldn't see the drill, but he would be aware of it going in, from the noise.

Monday, 6 June 2005

The nurses came to prepare Alan for the operation. He was taken to the theatre about mid-morning. I wasn't allowed to stay in the room because everything had to be disinfected. All the bed linen was changed, including mine, in readiness for his return.

I went for a walk in the grounds of the hospital. Large areas were neglected, although you could imagine that they had once been beautiful, and the whole hospital must have been a showcase for the old regime. Nevertheless, the grounds were still tranquil, and I found it therapeutic walking through them, to pass the time.

Michael went to the shops. He bought me a very useful laundry bowl, for my other therapy sessions, and at lunchtime he gave his English lesson.

The doctors and nurses wanted to improve their English and so those accompanying patients who were English-speaking, were 'invited' to give lessons. Michael wasn't keen to begin with. However, after a while, I think he almost started to enjoy it, and it was something to do during the long days with us. When he had to leave for home, they presented him with a lucky silk knot, as a gift, to say 'thank you'.

Eventually I had enough of the garden, so returned and sat outside the room. I wasn't allowed in, not until Alan came back. I tried to read one of the books I had brought with me for our stay, but I couldn't concentrate; thoughts and prayers were revolving round and round in my head. I almost wished I had been giving the English lesson for that day. What was Alan going through in the operating theatre? Would he be all right?

I must admit to praying that, if we couldn't have our miracle, Alan would die during surgery, so he could be spared the disease. I would be surprised if Alan didn't pray for the same.

The doors from the theatre opened. They were bringing Alan back. He looked cheerful and was wide awake. Michael was also back. His class had ended. Alan's first words, when we were all back in the room were, 'Needless to say, I have a very thick skull.' He had that wicked twinkle in his eyes that I had come to love so much. As always, he managed to break the ice and make us laugh. He told us how they had to reverse the drill, then go back in again, to get through his thick head! Thank God for his sense of humour.

One week later

Michael flew home. Alan was recovering well.

For the next two weeks, we followed the same routine, more or less. The routine started within a couple of days of the operation. Daily trips to the well-equipped gymnasium for physiotherapy sessions, would be added after about a week, but for the first week Alan was given a massage every morning, and at some point during the day, he received a visit from 'Dr. Pain' – our nickname for this individual because he administered an interesting technique.

He would enter the room with a broad grin, and begin mobilising Alan's arms, hands and fingers. Then he would do the same with his legs, feet and toes. With each movement he would ask, 'Pain?' at which Alan uttered the word 'Yes,' while trying to smile through contorted features, when he really wanted to say, 'You sadistic bugger.' Dr. Pain seemed happy with Alan's response. We assumed this was, at least in part, due to his being happy with Alan's progress. But we were not entirely convinced, because he spoke very little English. Perhaps he just enjoyed inflicting pain. We also believed he was trying to encourage messages between the part of the body he was moving and the brain. All I can say, for certain, was that he earned his nickname, and if his technique was designed to stimulate the nerves, it worked. Alan took it in good spirit, and was able to laugh. He was very brave.

Dr. Pain did show me a way of stimulating movement in the thumb, and an exercise to stretch the fingers, to try to keep them from curling under and stiffening into a permanent curled-up position. I continued to do all these things until the last month, or so, of Alan's life.

Saturday, 11 June 2005

The hospital driver took us to visit the Great Wall of China. Saturday and Sunday were meant to be his days off that week, but the hospital arranged for him to look after us, which he did happily, helped by the fee we paid him. We were fed up with being cooped-up in the hospital. It was good to get out, and the hospital driver was used to helping the patients, so he knew exactly what to do, which made it easier for me. I didn't take a camera to China. I hadn't expected to want to record anything, or make an album!

It was a long drive to the Great Wall. When we got there, the site was overrun with tourists. They streamed past countless stalls selling souvenirs, and we could see them all climbing up a segment of the Wall, to take in the views. We had a reasonable view from where we were, in the car park, so it was easier for us both to stay in the car and look at the wall winding away into the mountains and the breathtaking scenery, without having to fight the crowds.

Sunday, 12 June 2005

We set off late morning, for a second day of sightseeing. We had come to China to find a cure. We had not expected to find time to see the tourist sights. Yet we had seen Tian'anmen Square, the Great Wall, and we were on our way to see the Summer Palace, or the Garden of Perfect Purity, as the Chinese call it.

In a way, our trip to China made us feel like two intrepid explorers. It would be our last great adventure, and we had had quite a few since our first trip to Morocco in 1982. From the bobsleigh ride in St Moritz, to an amazing balloon flight in Kenya, when we had floated through the sky, undetected by the wildlife below. We came down so low over water that we could see the frogs on the leaves of the water lilies. There was the time we flew in a glider, and another time when we flew over active volcanoes, in a small seaplane. The latter had not been all that long ago, in 2002, when we went to New Zealand. The plane had seen better days, and I remembered how the control panel looked as though it was held together by sticking plaster. But nothing had depended on those adventures; not like our trip to China.

We were dropped off by the East Gate of the Summer Palace, by which most of the visitors enter. The storekeepers opposite the gates, helped the driver get Alan out of the car and into the wheelchair.

As I pushed Alan round the gardens, we tried to enjoy them, but it was difficult to appreciate what were indeed impressive grounds. They had been laid out by one of the emperors for his mother. A lake covers three quarters of the area of more than twelve square miles. There are areas shaded by trees, hills, bridges and pagodas. Lots of families were out for a Sunday stroll, all happily enjoying the afternoon. But we were both subdued. Had our trip been worth it? I am sure we were both asking ourselves the same question, but we never discussed it; not then, not afterwards. What was the point? For a short while we had been able to hope.

It was only when a storm started brewing overhead that we decided to make our way back to the car. The storekeepers helped get Alan back in, and we returned to the hospital.

Thursday, 16 June 2005

It was time to go home. The staff had been wonderful, and we were sad to be saying goodbye. We were sad for another reason as well. We tried to believe there was an improvement, but really there wasn't. By the time we got home, we had to admit to ourselves that Alan's condition had deteriorated. We felt despondent and low. We had failed to find our miracle.

Fighting the Disease

17 June 2005

It was good to be home. Or was it? What hope had we now? All we could do was make the best of it, and try to fight the disease. Easier said than done! Keeping up with it turned out to be an uphill battle all the way.

Alan's abilities were decreasing quite quickly which was something I never properly came to grips with. I continued to believe Alan could live for another three years, based on the prognosis we had been given. But there was never a moment to catch my breath, let alone take in what was happening before my eyes. I think Alan was aware of it, but I wasn't. All I noticed was the lack of respite or remission in an ever-downward spiral. I kept praying the disease would be slow but kind. It was neither slow nor kind, although it was kinder to us than many others.

It would have been kinder if it had been much quicker. I can see that now. But I was praying for quality time together, not for protracted suffering, and that is what it was – protracted suffering.

In the months that followed, I often felt as though we were under siege from all directions. Whenever we tried to do something to improve our situation, it usually got sabotaged. If it wasn't the disease that stopped us from living the way we wanted, it was health and safety regulations. If it wasn't this, then it was inadequate information and support. Finally, when it came to dying, after all the humiliation of the disease, the law in this country – devoid of compassion – denied Alan the right to choose to die at home, when his life became unbearable for him.

Alan had an exit plan. Why didn't he decide to go to Switzerland for an assisted suicide, when we got back from China? If he had been given a choice, it might have been to die then, while he still had some dignity. But he would have chosen to die at home, not in another country.

Besides, after China, Switzerland was no longer a straightforward choice, because Alan would now need to be accompanied. Anyone who accompanied him risked the possibility of prosecution, on returning to this country. He would not have wanted to put me under that pressure, or have risked me being prosecuted for taking him. He couldn't put me through that. While we could have discussed this together a year or so before, now it was difficult for me to broach the subject, not because I was afraid of prosecution, but because I felt that if I raised the subject, it might seem to him that I was putting him under pressure to go; that he was a burden I didn't want. I didn't want him to think that, and I wanted him to live for as long as he wanted to live. If, on one day, he said that he wanted to die, I took it to be a bad day. Everyone has bad days. Only if he made it really apparent that he wanted to die would I have taken him at his word. Eventually he did.

It was my job to make sure he knew how much I loved him, and keep him as comfortable as I could for as long as he wanted to go on living. But I often failed under the strain. I realise now, that for both of us, the idea of losing each other was always going to be as painful as living with the disease. Going to Switzerland would not be an easy decision for him to make in the end. If he had been given the choice of being assisted to die at home, he would probably have left it until he found life intolerable, or about to become so. Eventually it was, but the law would not spare him the humiliation and suffering, and give him the right to die in dignity at home, at the time of his choosing. I will never know whether he lived with the disease for a lot longer than he would have chosen or how much he put up with unbearable suffering because of the laws of this country. Thinking back on the months after the operation, I can only liken it to living in a war zone. In war, you have virtually no control over your life. Nothing is certain. Your freedom is taken from you. This is the way it was for us. We were trapped, and over the coming months we would find ourselves fighting battles on several fronts. I can think of at least three. The first was my being able to meet Alan's needs, without going under myself. The second was trying to meet both our needs, as opposed to what other people appeared to demand of us. The third was the most hopeless of all. Yet it was the one which I most wanted to win. It was the battle to prevent the cruel effects of Motor Neurone Disease. Everyday, there was some torture I had to watch Alan endure, some humiliation I was unable to prevent. I felt angry with anyone who threatened my ability to protect him, and even more angry with those who made it harder.

I don't think Alan felt intolerable physical discomfort, not until the end. But I am sure he felt mental pain and humiliation. The torment for us both was particularly the humiliation. A method often used by torturers is to think through all the permutations of mental pain. They use their power to humiliate their victim, to torment them mentally, and let other people witness it. That is what the disease did to us.

Many stood by and did nothing, either through ignorance, or because they lacked the backup. But many were very kind and often kindness came from the most unexpected sources. Had it been other wise, I would almost certainly have lost faith in the human race.

One day, not long after Alan died, I met a man at a bus stop in Barnes, on my way to London. He was a recent refugee from Afghanistan. He was eighty years old, a professor, and apparently spoke many languages. His father had been a government minister in the days of the old monarchy. His closest family had been tortured in front of him, by the Taliban. He was a Muslim, but had come to this country because he believed its Christian values would result in compassion for his plight.

The only help he had encountered since his arrival, was from a Sikh. In exchange for some household duties, the Sikh had given him a roof over his head. His possessions amounted to the clothes he wore, and I assume a little money. He washed out his clothes each night, before bed, and left them to dry, ready for the next day. He wasn't looking for charity. He simply wanted to be given respect, understanding and compassion. I couldn't fail to notice the pain he felt. As he related his story to me, tears welled up in his eyes. I felt such a strong empathy with him that tears came to mine. He was disappointed and angry and clearly felt let down. I felt the same. He had lost the people he loved in a cruel way. I had lost Alan in a cruel way. He was alone. I was alone. I wished I could have taken his pain away, just as I wished someone would take away mine.

9 July 2005

Days out with Alan were becoming more difficult, which was the reason he insisted I went to The Hampton Court Flower Show with my mother. We had gone the previous year together and he didn't want to spoil that memory with one of me pushing him round in a wheelchair. His golfing friend, George, came over to stay with him. I couldn't leave him on his own for lengthy periods any more as he was unable to do very much with his hands by now, and could barely press the button on the alarm device for Helpline. I would have to sort something out very quickly, but I didn't know what.

Serendipity, rather than organised outside help, played its part in solving the problem. The equipment for Helpline was due for a check, and the person who came told me about environmental control systems. She gave me the name of a company, which I telephoned straight away. I thought we would have to pay for such a system to be installed, but from what she described it would be worth it. However, when I telephoned the company, Possum Controls Limited, they felt we should be able to get it through the NHS. They started the ball rolling and made contact for me. I am forever grateful to them.

Before China, we coped with limited support from carers, social services and the hospice. We preferred it that way, so we could maintain some privacy and control over our lives. We wanted to do so for as long as possible. But after China, we really couldn't do without assistance in a variety of forms. Our need would become ever greater.

In order to enable Alan to stay at home, major alterations to the house were needed. It was also clear that we needed a specially adapted mobility vehicle as I was finding it extremely difficult to get Alan in and out of the car on my own.

Before we made the decision on a suitable vehicle, the hospice occupational therapist recommended that we should go to an assessment centre, where we would be given advice on a suitable vehicle, or modifications to a vehicle. Incidentally, I had no idea that we should have had access to the social services' occupational therapists. The hospice staff tried their best to give us the information we needed but they were better trained to help people suffering from cancer and had little experience of the needs of someone with MND.

When I contacted the vehicle assessment centre, I was told there was a long waiting list. I can't remember how long, but it was too long for us, given the rate of progression of the disease. So Alan and I made our own assessment and found a company that could supply what we considered we would need. The company brought a vehicle to the house, to give us a demonstration, and this enabled us to make our final decision. That was it, decision made. We were fortunate that we were able to afford to do this. I was beginning to learn that assessment was another word for delay or, worse, not happening at all. How could this make life bearable for a person suffering from a cruel terminal illness? How could it make them feel less of a burden?

The van, as I christened it, had a ramp, so I could push Alan onto it in the wheelchair. The wheelchair was secured alongside me. It was as near to a normal driving experience as we could get, while protecting my back. We tried everything to maintain some normality in our relationship. We wanted to remain a couple. But it was becoming harder and harder. The van allowed us to stay independently mobile – Alan had a decent view of the road ahead, and we could converse easily when we wanted to. It gave us the freedom of going out on our own together, and we didn't have to wait for others to drive Alan here, there and everywhere. There was always the risk that he would be tempted to tell me how to drive. He had been inclined to do this in the past; the reason he did most of the driving, before he was ill.

He had loved driving. It was the reason his daughter's birthday present to him one year, had been a racing day at Brands Hatch; the chance to drive a racing car. However, to his credit, he rarely told me how to drive, once I had to do it all. The only situation in which he would say anything was if he felt we might be about to have an accident, which was fair enough. I knew stress could and did affect the quality of my driving, so instead of being annoyed, I appreciated his intervention. He handled it extremely well.

We were also lucky that the van took the much larger wheelchair, which Alan would come to need in the latter months of his life. Another bit of serendipity. He would need a wheelchair with a back that could tilt him into a reclined position. This rested his head back for him, and, took the strain off the muscles supporting it. Eventually, these muscles would become too weak for him to keep his head up by himself, and this would affect his ability to breathe comfortably and speak, because his larynx would be squashed. It was my mother who knew what to do to make him more comfortable. Her nursing experience and knowledge continued to prove useful. She noticed why he was having difficulty, and generally came up with a solution. I was usually too busy fighting fires, being the 'doer', and I didn't have her knowledge or experience. The physiotherapists came up with ideas as well, and Alan had his own, of course. Between us we kept him physically comfortable most of the time, but it was an uphill battle. What would work one day wouldn't work the next.

27 July 2005

The doctor came to assess Alan for the environmental control system. A visitor from the NHS had already been to see us and explained that, because Alan had MND, he could be 'fast-tracked', and for that same reason, we wouldn't have to pay for the equipment. Means-testing was not required. This was a first for us, and music to our ears. At the very first meeting for the system, we were told we had fallen upon one of the best kept secrets of the NHS. Why a secret, when people have such a real need for it?

Protocol required their doctor to make the assessment, and confirm the need, before we would have the go-ahead. This was apparently just a formality, because Alan had MND.

8 September 2005

The environmental control system started to be installed. It took a couple of visits to set it up, and over the coming months it would need adjustments to meet Alan's changing abilities. From the first meeting to installation took approximately two months, which was fast compared to everything else we encountered. Installation was reasonably easy. It requires very little wiring, provided one has enough electric sockets, and few were required. The most complicated part was wiring the front door, to enable Alan to open it. He could do this remotely, without moving from the riser/recliner chair – the chair that had been loaned to us by the MND Association. This was now the most comfortable (and safest) place for him to be during the day, and it helped him stand up when necessary. An intercom was fitted, so he could ask who was at the door, before triggering the system to unlock it.

The system meant that it didn't matter if I lost my keys or was held up. He could open the door on his own, without the risk of leaving his chair. And, by pressing a pad behind his head, he was able to select from a variety of options. Once again he could make telephone calls on his own, call for help by activating the telephone line to Helpline, or summon me if I was nearby. When I was working in the garden, or in another part of the house, I had a bleeper with me, which would sound. It gave us both more freedom, for a while at least. It gave him some quality of life and the ability to make some choices without reference to others.

Alan could choose which channel he wanted to watch, without having to get someone to turn the television over for him. My command of the remote was short lived, but it was worth it!

I was beginning to realise how little understanding or empathy some people have with disability. There was a bright spark who dropped by one day soon after the environmental control system was installed. I don't know if she was trying to make a light-hearted remark. She said: 'well, at least you can watch TV, and you've got a roof over your head. What more can you want?' I don't know what made her say it. Why did she have to say anything? Her remarks made us both angry, frustrated and sad all at the same time.

The system together with a computer would allow him to access the internet, and make it possible for him to read books and newspapers. At a later stage, with the necessary software, he could also use it to communicate. As I indicated earlier, Alan was a bit of a technophobe, as far as computers were concerned. Furthermore, he had always been physically active. He was never going to find this an easy or desirable way to overcome some of the difficulties of the disease.

Life revolved around the illness, and organising everything to overcome the difficulties it caused, or might cause in the future. After China, the effect of having little me-time, and being helpless to prevent the deterioration, started to take its toll. The building work for the alterations to the house, whilst essential, didn't help. It wasn't as though we were doing it so we could both enjoy the results.

The first time I reacted badly to the effect of the disease was the evening I decided to do a chocolate pudding for dessert. Whenever we had it, Alan ate it, but it was not his favourite. I knew this, but I felt like a comfort pudding that evening, and it was one of my favourites. Not any more though, not after this! As I served his up, he announced 'I don't want chocolate pudding!' The way he said it was selfish, and even slightly childish. It made me annoyed. I shouted, 'Well I do!' and threw his across the room. The pudding caught his shoulder, just before it hit the fridge door. The mess was terrible. For the first few seconds, it was worth it. It was worth it for the release of tension. But then I was ashamed of myself. Alan was crying, sobbing. We had been warned that emotional lability, either laughing or crying inappropriately, was a symptom of the disease. But it wasn't the reason he was crying on this occasion. I had made him cry, because I had shown the strain I was under. He felt it was his fault, and he was helpless to stop it.

Before, I had hated the disease for what it was doing to Alan. Now I hated it for what it was beginning to do to me. I couldn't keep the strain to myself. Yet being cross with him was the last thing I wanted. In the past, it hadn't mattered if I got cross with him; he got cross with me. That's what couples do. But it would matter from then on, because he had a cruel terminal illness, and I wanted to avoid getting annoyed with him. To help myself avoid this, I would attempt to put myself in his shoes. The times when I couldn't do so were generally the times when I was simply too tired, and sadly, I showed my irritation. Sometimes he did seem demanding, but then the frustrations he must have been feeling would have been enormous. At least I could do things for myself, even if I had too much to do. He handled his frustration incredibly well. I could not always handle the effects of the disease as well he did.

21 September 2005

Social services visited; the same young woman who had been to see us all those months back when I had flu. I had been in touch with her to request the visit. After China the disease was clearly gaining the upper hand. It was overwhelming, emotionally and physically. The strain was becoming all too apparent. The chocolate pudding incident frightened me. I had never behaved in this way before.

She spent two hours going through everything with us. How the illness was already impacting on our lives and my ability to look after Alan. I was told I could leave our worries with her. She would come back to me with some recommendations and ideas. I was told: 'That is what we are here for.' I am not good at delegating, and find it especially difficult to leave important matters to someone else. However, I was tired and grateful for any assistance. I did as she suggested, and waited for her to come back to me, for the time being at least.

We were not asking for any financial assistance. Because we were not in a position to qualify for any means-tested help, I didn't think we were entitled to any. We were fortunate, but we – and in particular Alan – had worked hard to be in this position. I can't help feeling that he deserved more help than was offered. However, at the time I was simply grateful for any assistance that came our way, and I remain glad that we could afford what we did. However, as a result of the visit, I was awarded vouchers by social services – vouchers that could be used towards respite costs to help the carer.

Although financial help was useful, it was not what I was looking for primarily. I was hoping for information, advice and someone to organise anything that could make life easier. I was led to believe and I needed to believe, this would be forthcoming. I knew I couldn't last a lengthy battle without additional troops.

Alan and I had these meetings and conversations many times over, with various professionals who came to see us over the forthcoming months. We told them about the physical and mental effects. The words always fell on sympathetic ears. They genuinely wanted to know how we were getting on, and what they could do to help. If I knew, I told them. For the most part, however, it might as well have fallen on deaf ears. We needed the kind of support given to a lot of dying cancer patients who choose to die at home. We needed to know how to access nursing and carer support, together with the equipment required for the job. Sadly, for a long time, we did not receive this level of assistance, and by the time it started to happen it was too late.

I often felt as though I was playing the same old gramophone record. I might just as well have recorded one of these meetings, and put the tape on each time anyone came to see us. On reflection, I could have used the hours better just by spending time and talking with Alan. It makes me think of that poem by William Henry Davies, *'What is life if, full of care, We have no time to stand and stare …'*

Of course, Alan had plenty of time in the day, but we couldn't spend it together, not in the way we had in the past. Looking after his basic needs and comfort always took precedence over everything else, including those all-important hugs. Alan couldn't hug me; I could still hug him. But life was often too fraught. He must have wanted a hug at times, just as much as I did.

I always hoped there would be some point in these meetings. I hoped we would have time for each other at the end of Alan's life. I hoped we would have time when we would not be fighting battles on all fronts. We had already lost the battle to defy the disease.

But we never got this time. Instead, Alan looked on helplessly as I became more and more tired and distraught, as I teetered on the edge of depression or behaved like a raving lunatic. For most of the last months of Alan's life, he must have wondered what would happen to him if I went under. Indeed, I wondered the same. The only thing that kept me from going absolutely mad was the knowledge that he needed me to look after him. Even in my worst moments, and I had many, no one could have cared for him as I did.

11 October 2005

Alan went into the hospice for a week, to give me respite. I didn't like it any more than he did, but I was exhausted, and had to have a break. I will always be grateful for this support and I am not sure where I would have been without it. Social services still hadn't come back to me. It had been three weeks since they had been to see us. Three weeks is a very long time for a disease like MND. I was getting more and more exhausted and frightened that I would not cope – that there would be more incidents like the chocolate pudding.

After three weeks of waiting, I made several attempts to speak to our social worker. She was rarely in the office, and appeared to be extremely stretched, so eventually I managed to speak to her line manager. I was desperate. My voice must have conveyed near-hysteria. Finally, some action! They would get us assessed for continuing care. This would put us in the system and mean that the NHS might pay or contribute to Alan's ever increasing care needs. It was welcome action, but I did not know when the assessment would be made, nor did it recognise the urgency of my immediate need for help. No one seemed to have any real idea of the impact of this disease, and the need to be able to act quickly. I had to be desperate, to be begging for help, before anything happened. It was humiliating. Alan understood. It was as if they were the grown-ups giving a forlorn child a pat on the head and a 'there,

there'. After this, they expect you to t carry on as though nothing is wrong. But I couldn't. It would make me angry, very angry. It seemed so cruel.

Getting adequate support was something I battled with to the very end. We had been able to manage, until this time, with one carer who came each morning to help me get Alan up, except for Sunday. We tried to keep Sunday completely free of people, for as long as we could. It was very tiring, having a continual stream of visitors, even though they were there to help, or trying to, and it was always a difficult balancing act, maintaining privacy versus having sufficient help. On Sunday, we liked to be able to stay in bed, and get up late. I had to read the papers to Alan, once he couldn't hold or turn the pages of the newspaper for himself, but we liked this time to ourselves.

On the days when we had a carer, they got Alan bathed and dressed. They came at 10.30 in the morning, after I had given Alan his physiotherapy exercises and breakfast. After China, Alan was able to do very few exercises without assistance. His legs remained strong for some time, possibly as a result of his cycling days,. Alan had his physiotherapy sessions twice a week, and the physiotherapists showed me the exercises for me to do with him, on the other days. This way we hoped to maintain the strength in his muscles and mobility in his joints. Gradually, as he could do less and less, I had to do more and more. My morning sessions with him got longer and longer. Although I found it exhausting, it was something positive to fight the disease, and we managed to make some fun from these sessions as well. Lying on his back, with his knees bent up, his feet would be pressed against my stomach. I would kneel on the bed and he pushed as hard as he could, stopping before he forced me off the bed –just before, which made us laugh. Alan was determined to maintain the strength in his muscles, and whether or not it was because of these exercises, he was still able to stand until two weeks before he died.

In addition to the morning call, a carer came in for a couple of hours during the day, two days a week. This meant, I was able to do things like the shopping on one of the days. On the other day, I did my one-day-a-week voluntary work with the gardening charity. Alan had a massage that day, so between this and the carer, I could just about cover the time I was out working. I say working, but in reality it was the best respite I could have had. The garden still had the power to revive me. There was half an hour to an hour before I got home, when he was on his own. He liked to have this time with no one around, and the environmental control system allowed him to manage, for the time being.

On a Wednesday, Alan went to the day centre at the hospice. These few hours of not having to keep an eye on him or organise someone to do it for me, enabled me to catch up on paperwork, organise anything needed for him and, with a bit of luck, clean the house. It was originally suggested that this could be my 'me day.' Perhaps I would like to have a massage or some other form of pampering? Nice thought in an ideal world!

Mid-Late October 2005

Alan was now restricted to the wheelchair when we went out. In the house he still used the walker, and he wanted to continue standing and walking, albeit with this aid, for as long as he could. Deep down, I knew that once he could no longer walk, or more particularly stand, I had lost him. He had said it himself, 'Once my trunk has gone that's it'. He could live without the use of his arms and hands - that took great courage and acceptance, but the day his trunk went, the parts of the disease he dreaded most would soon follow. For as long as he could stand and walk he knew he still had muscles supporting his spine. Once his trunk was gone, life wouldn't be worth living.

But when we went out, we had to use a wheelchair. It really

wasn't practical to do anything else. So Alan wanted one he could operate himself. It would give him more freedom and save me having to
push. Pushing up a hill is hard work, and everything we did these days
seemed like pushing the wheelchair uphill. He was thinking of me, as
well as himself. Our MND Association Visitor told me to get in touch
with their Regional Care Development Advisor who might be able to
give us some advice, and maybe some financial assistance.

I made contact, and was told that first of all I had to get Wheelchair Services to assess Alan. A decision as to how best to help, would
be based on that assessment. And so there was another wait for an assessment!

End October 2005

From the end of October, a carer came for half an hour at night,
for two or three nights per week. This was in addition to the morning
call. It was all the additional help I was able to organise, because there
weren't enough carers available for the other nights. Nevertheless, for
two or three days a week I now had help to get Alan up and dressed in
the morning, and to get him to bed.

Over the coming months, the company, that provided our carers
tried their best to increase their capacity. In the last month of Alan's life,
we had two carers who came twice in the morning. The first call was a
short, half-hour visit to take him to the toilet. They came back a second
time, mid-morning, after exercises and breakfast, in order to get him up,
showered and dressed. This gave me time to get myself washed and
ready for the day ahead. At night, we had two carers to put Alan to bed.

In reality, I needed this support sooner, but it took time for the
care company to recruit additional carers to make it possible. Even then
continuity was a very real problem. Lack of continuity didn't help Alan,
because what he could do one week he couldn't do the next. When the
carer changed, it meant that what he needed had to be explained all over

again, and this wasn't easy for him especially when speech became more of a problem. And it didn't help me, because I would end up showing them what to do, or explaining on Alan's behalf, thus defeating the object of having the help. Having carers coming in, was the only way to look after Alan at home, other than having full-time live-in care. That was something we both wanted to avoid, because of the level of intrusion it would mean. Already, it was hard to get quality time on our own.

And Alan tried really hard to make it as easy as possible for me. He would use his wonderful sense of humour to make light of difficulties, and he would put his mind to thinking of the best way to do something, because he knew I didn't have time to think. The gradient in front of our daily slog was feeling steeper and steeper, like pushing the wheelchair uphill.

Mid-November 2005

We were assessed for continuing care and soon after, I received a telephone call, to let me know that we had failed the criteria. After I put the phone down, I thought about this decision and wondered what on earth would make us fit the criteria. However, we were now in the system, so it would be quicker to get reassessed, whenever it was felt to be appropriate. Why it was not appropriate at this point, I don't know. People with lesser physical needs managed to qualify. It is supposed to be based on a health need. I think it was because Alan was well-cared-for, which was only because I couldn't leave him any other way, and I appeared to be in control. It was easier for them to look at the thin exterior layer. I gave them an excuse to do nothing. The house was clean, Alan was cared for, and I tried to make sure he was comfortable, so no one wanted to look beneath the surface.

I made many pleas for help to those who should have been able to help. Some help made it through the increasing levels of bombardment from the disease. I grasped any hand I saw through the smoke of the battlefield.

There were those, outside the care system, who helped us in many unexpected ways: mainly friends and people that Alan and I had known for many years. Sometimes people came to stay with Alan, like George had when I went to the flower show; friends made and delivered a fish pie, one of Alan's favourite meals; others came and took him out for lunch. Lunch with the boys brought a little normality back to his life. And, knowing that he was both in company he enjoyed and good hands, meant I could have a real break. Most importantly, Michael would come over and spend time with his father. He did odd jobs for me around the house, at the same time. They were jobs his father would have done, had he been able. I appreciated this a great deal, but not simply because of what it meant to me. It meant an enormous amount to Alan. He felt he was able to do something for me, if only through his son.

Some people really did go to a lot of trouble, either to make things possible, or to make them easier, or both.

The dentist used to completely rearrange his surgery, so Alan could have his check-ups, at the same time as his hygienist appointment, and in the same room. Although Alan had started to find it more diffi-cult, he had persevered at cleaning his own teeth, until we got back from China. After China, the carers and I had to clean them for him, but I also increased the visits to the hygienist. I didn't want Alan to get one of the infections he had been so prone to acquiring in the past. Our dentist made it as easy as possible for us. He even used to push Alan in and out of the van for me!

The hairdresser came up with ingenious ways of washing Alan's hair. It was easier for all concerned, if he stayed in the wheelchair, so a bucket of water was held behind his head to wash his hair. Sitting in the wheelchair, he couldn't get his head over the wash basin. This way, we kept up appointments at the hairdresser until a very short time before he died. Again, a little bit of normality. He also enjoyed the pampering, and it was a different way to pass the time. I stayed with him, and was treated to cups of coffee and magazines while I waited for him, so we both had an outing.

On one occasion, my sister made the journey from her home in Kent, just to clean the house for me. She came, worked like a Trojan and went back –all on the same day. Not having enough time to do it myself used to get me down. Both Alan and I had always been very tidy people, and if the house was in order I felt more in control. I could have had someone to come and clean for me, but that would have been someone else in the house, and with so many people coming in and out of our lives everyday, it was very difficult to achieve any privacy. And it only got worse, as the disease progressed.

24 November 2005

Alan had a meeting at Pedigree Group. He was still a director of this company, having been part of the original management consortium that bought Pedigree Toys and Dolls, as it was known in the 1980s. Every couple of months all the directors tried to get together for a meeting. Even at this late stage, Alan attended. I would drive him to those meetings and stay with him, in case he needed help with things like looking at papers, as he couldn't turn the pages.

When they bought the company, it had a lot of problems, but its one great strength was the teenage doll brand, Sindy. They hoped to capitalise on this, and in time use it to develop the company into other product areas.

Alan had been instrumental in putting together the advertising and promotional plans, which would support the relaunch of Sindy. They were presented to the sales force and retail buyers, at the London Hippodrome. I was in the audience, and felt very much a part of it, not least because Alan and I had had many discussions about the plans over our kitchen table. During our working lives, we had often sought each other's advice, and as I had just successfully relaunched Old Spice, at the time, I was able to provide some useful input. When he stood on stage to give his presentation, he made me feel so proud. He had looked especially dashing in his new suit, and the tie I had bought him for luck.

The plans Alan presented were not without risk. Hence, the Finance Director had described the event as "one big party to add another zero" to the potential losses they could make. But the risk paid off and Alan remained a Director, even after he retired from Parlour Wood. He enjoyed it. As he had put it to me one day, with a little wicked laughter, 'I can make suggestions and recommendations in the knowledge that I will not be the poor bugger who will have to implement them!'

I enjoyed helping him during these meetings, and because I was there, the directors would involve me, by asking me for my opinions. It was like the old days, when we had shared our thoughts and ideas about our work; an opportunity to do something together; something which had nothing to do with the disease. These meetings became respite for us both. A chance to do something normal, and be with friends and colleagues, rather than people associated with the disease.

We were both determined to try to keep our lives as normal as possible for as long as we could. We would still go out for lunch on our own, for as long as I was able to manage alone. We still went shopping together for some things, and Alan enjoyed helping me choose things for the garden. He also quite enjoyed going to gardens with me.

None of these things could replace golf, of course. Nothing could. We both knew that, so we didn't talk about it. What was the point?

5 December 2005

The shower room downstairs still wasn't ready. We had been waiting for months for the floor to dry out. Once it was dry enough to lay the non-slip floor covering, we discovered the pipework had been installed incorrectly. It was the last thing I needed. It was getting more and more difficult to get Alan in and out of the bath upstairs. I could see that we were going to need to use the shower room very soon. Here I was, fighting like hell to keep Alan at home, and again I felt as though all my efforts were being sabotaged.

All the floor-boards on the landing had to come up. It was apparently the simplest way to solve the problem, but it was exactly what I had tried to avoid, for fear of Alan tripping and falling. I made my feelings known. The plumber seemed to have no idea why I was so upset. But it was Alan and I who would have to bear the brunt, emotionally and physically - not him. Fortunately, the builder backed me up, and I only had one disgruntled workman to deal with, not two.

9 December 2005

Wheelchair Services finally came to assess Alan's wheelchair. We were expecting them to give us advice about one which he could operate himself, one with some support for his head. He couldn't hold his head up easily now. It was straining the muscles, and he had to let it fall forward. This had become particularly apparent over the last week.

He had to use the wheelchair to go out for his birthday lunch with his golf friends. We were still using the wheelchair we had been using since China. He was sitting in it for a long time with his head unsupported.

This can't have helped his neck muscles. I was angry, and even more so when they told us that, because he couldn't hold his head up, it wouldn't be safe for him to operate his own chair. I felt Alan's frustration.

I didn't know enough about wheelchairs to know what was suitable. It wasn't like making the decision over the 'van'. That was why we needed an assessment. But it had taken so long; too long for a disease like MND. Even now, there was a lot of deliberation over what would be suitable.

12 December 2005

We went to the Royal Brompton Hospital for a sleep test. The pipework for the shower room was being done while we were there. The visit to the Brompton had been suggested by Alan's neurologist, because they specialise in helping people with respiratory disorders. It would help us to get some measure of how well Alan's respiratory muscles were working. Monitors would be put on him, before he went to sleep, to measure the levels of oxygen and carbon dioxide in his lungs. The test meant a stay in hospital of up to five days.

Hospital visits were a necessary evil, and the ones to King's and the Brompton required quite a lot of effort, although the latter was easier, and it could have been made even easier.

There wasn't any overnight parking at the hospital, and no one had told me that I could have requested an ambulance to take us there and back, not until we were at the hospital! So I had to drop Alan off and leave him, which I didn't like, while I took the van and my mother back to her home. I was grateful that my mother had come with us to help me to settle Alan into our room, and that she lived close enough for me to do this, otherwise I am not sure what I would have done.

While I went to park the car, the hospital organised a 'put-you-up' bed in the room, for me. As in China, we had our own room, with its own bathroom. But in a way, it wasn't as comfortable. There wasn't as much light, but other than this I can't say why it didn't seem as comfortable, and it is possible my impression of it may have been coloured by the way I was feeling at the time.

This stay, like his other times in hospital, didn't give me any faith in the ability of hospital staff to look after Alan properly. I was glad I was with him, because the nurses didn't seem to know what to do. One of the nurses remarked that she was glad that I was there. They wanted to look after him properly, and I had been able to guide them. But how would he have been looked after, if I had not been there?

The visit was worth the effort. They didn't only do the sleep test. The staff advised us on how we might control some of the symptoms Alan could suffer through not being able to breathe effectively. The symptoms include tiredness, headaches and even hallucinations and nightmares. They occur through a build-up of carbon dioxide in the lungs. Other problems include choking and difficulty clearing saliva, as the muscles in the throat weaken.

In an emergency, or for short-term situations, an invasive procedure is sometimes performed, called a tracheostomy*. However, in Alan's case the hospital recommended Non-invasive Positive Pressure Ventilation (NPPV). It doesn't suit everyone, and the user needs to be able to coordinate their breathing with the ventilator machine. However, it had the potential to make life more bearable, should Alan start to suffer any problems. We were told it would be less likely than a tracheostomy, to extend Alan's life beyond the point when he no longer wanted to live. He could stop using it whenever he chose and there were other ways as well to make him comfortable from the symptoms he might suffer at a later stage. We did not cover these, at this point. I didn't think to ask. Alan's sleep test result showed his oxygen levels were virtually normal, so the time when we would need to know these things seemed some way off. We could ask at our next visit.

We were sent away with an NPPV machine and masks to try. I was given one quick lesson just before we left the hospital, and was told I could phone the hospital, should I need further guidance. I have to admit that I was terrified that Alan would need it before our next visit, which would not be for another three months. I felt far from confident about using the equipment.

Machines are fine, if you know what you are doing with them.

But when you don't, or are afraid they might go wrong, then they become very intimidating. I had to adapt quickly to a lot of changes. Some I found easier than others. But I never came to grips with the speed at which I was being required to adapt emotionally or physically to the disease.

The information and support we were given during our stay was more useful than much of what we had received from others. The medical staff used the opportunity to talk to Alan about how he might manage other problems he could meet with the disease, such as difficulty with swallowing and getting sufficient nourishment. They showed him different types of feeding tubes. Although this was something we didn't want to think about, we knew that we might have to eventually. Then there was the wheelchair: because it had not been sorted out before we went to the hospital, we had resorted to putting a board behind Alan's back, and holding his head back against it with a long scarf. This held his head up for him. We wrapped the scarf round his forehead and then tied it behind the board. We improvised. We often had to improvise. But the hospital was horrified that we had been forced to come up with this as make-do-and-mend solution. They were horrified that Alan did not have a suitable wheelchair. They got onto Wheelchair Services to chase them on our behalf.

And that was not all: the hospital's occupational therapist asked me what equipment support I had at home. That was a joke. For at least two months I had been trying to organise ceiling hoists, but had been getting little more than negative advice - what would not be suitable, rather than what would be. A bit like the wheelchair! In fact I had become so disenchanted with the advice I was getting, and desperate, that I had resorted to doing it myself, as usual. I got a private company who supplied hoists, to advise us. I had not long placed the order. I did have a mobile hoist, which the hospice had organised, but in theory it needed two people to operate it. It was certainly heavy and unwieldy to push around.

This hoist had finally been loaned to us, because one day, at the very end of November, I had screamed down the telephone to a member of staff at the hospice. I still feel angry at having been reduced to this state, a state of utter desperation. And it had to happen so many times, in order for anything to be done. And I feel angrier, when I think about the effect this must have had on Alan.

The frustrations arising from watching someone you love dying from a hopeless, terminal illness, are immense. Add to this the daily, and ever-increasing frustrations of meeting opposition and lack of action, on virtually every front. I would reach a point when I felt as though my head would implode and I had to scream out loud. If I had not screamed, I think I would have gone mad. There were moments when I probably was near to madness, and there were many times, in the latter part of Alan's life, when I was reduced to screaming. I wish it had not been so, because it upset him a great deal to see me this way, just as it upset me to see what the disease was doing to him. I felt helpless in all my attempts to make things any better.

The Brompton hospital told us that we should have been entitled to hoists via the social services without having to be means tested, without having to order them myself. Furthermore, when they saw what we had to cope with: the effect of the disease on Alan's abilities, they couldn't understand why Alan had not been entitled to Continuing Care at the recent assessment.

For a brief moment, I felt relief. Here were people who understood what we were up against, prepared to give us some ammunition, and even to do a little bit of fighting on our behalf. But it was brief and had come incredibly late. We would never be able to make up the time.

Just before Christmas 2005

Thanks to the Brompton, a more suitable and comfortable wheelchair suddenly materialised. Happy Christmas! We still needed to use the head scarf, to hold Alan's head back against the headrest when the chair wasn't in a reclined position. But at least it reclined, and at least it had a headrest. It was also easier to push than the previous one.

Christmas 2005

Somehow, I had done the cards and posted them, got the presents and wrapped them, and bought the tree and dressed it. I had done everything I always did, to get ready for Christmas. I wanted it to be happy. I wanted it to be normal, well as normal as it could be –this was likely to be our last Christmas. I don't know to what extent I realised this at the time. Based on what we had been told at King's, we could still have years, but something was telling me that this was not likely. So I wish it could have been a happier Christmas. But instead it turned out to be one of those times when you want to rewind the tape and edit out or change the bits you don't like.

My mother came to stay, and we took everyone, that is Michael and his family, Caroline and her family, my mother and even, Valerie, Alan's wife, so that she could be with her children and grandchildren, out to a local restaurant on Christmas Eve, everything as usual. I was looking forward to a quiet Christmas Day, a day to cherish as a special day with Alan, without the whole family. We were both tired after the hospital, and everything else that had happened in the lead up to Christmas.

On Christmas day, we were expecting to see Alan's son and his family as they said they would just pop in on their way to the Midlands. Michael's wife wanted to spend part of Christmas day with her family. We were looking forward to them coming. We hadn't seen them on a Christmas day before - they had always been in Australia.

But everyone turned up, Michael with his family, Caroline with hers, and their mother as well. I think I would have been able to cope with this unexpected invasion, if she had not come as well, but in my frazzled state, Valerie being there was too much.

I couldn't see why she had to come; just as I couldn't see why she used to come to sit with Alan on the days when I was at the gardening charity. She would come for an hour, instead of Caroline, to cover the period before I got home, when I couldn't leave Alan alone any more, even for short periods. He didn't want a carer to be organised, if at all possible. Of course, he preferred the company of his daughter to a stranger, but his wife came more often than not. Alan had left his wife more than thirty years before. It was his daughter he wanted to see, not his wife. Why did she come instead? It did not occur to me then, but reflecting back on these moments, it more than likely had something to do with the fact that she had never properly let go. At the time when I was most vulnerable, she was staking her claim.

Everything was different that Christmas. Not only was I was losing all that I loved; all that I loved was also being defiled by the disease. His children were with us, and it should have made me happy. I know they wanted to make the day special for their father. They brought mulled wine to heat up in the kitchen and nibbles. But how could they understand?

It didn't help that we were not asked, or that we were not expecting his wife, although it wasn't unusual for her to come to a family gathering, or to turn up unannounced.

Suddenly, it all became too much. I sat down on the sofa next to where Alan was, in his chair, and started to cry. I just wanted to be alone with him then. He looked at me as if to say, 'I wish I could do something.' But he couldn't. Instead, Alan's wife came over. She sat down on the sofa beside me, and put an arm around me. I think she meant well, simply trying to console me, but it was probably the worst thing that could have happened. Out of all the people in the house, including my own mother, it had to be Valerie who put an arm round me. Why? The disease seemed to be taunting me.

Of course, the person I desperately needed to put their arms around me was Alan. But he was helpless. Only he could come close to understanding what I felt at that moment, and that what had happened had made it worse, but he was helpless.

So I let her console me, for a short time. Then I made my excuses, and went upstairs to the bathroom, on the pretence that I needed to dry my eyes. But I needed to escape. I had done this when I was growing up to escape family arguments. As I sat there on the toilet seat, on Christmas Day, all those feelings of vulnerability, insecurity and isolation that I had experienced back then, which Alan had expelled, returned. In fact, they had been gradually creeping back, one by one, ever since we returned from China. When I was growing up the bathroom had been my sanctuary. From now on, it would become my sanctuary again. It was a place to hide from the impact of the disease. I would often need to escape the disease, but I suppose I was lucky I could; Alan couldn't.

Perhaps, if I hadn't been so tired by Christmas Day, it might have been different. I couldn't say. For that time, when they were all with us, I felt like an intruder in my own home. Increasingly, I had felt like an intruder, and this feeling would only get worse. Home was feeling less like home, all the time.

After they went, Mum suggested we open our presents. Alan looked grateful that she was trying to lighten the atmosphere, and make me feel better.

He had managed to organise some presents for me. I think his son had bought one or two of them, on his behalf. They were things I had mentioned I would like during the course of the year, things which

Alan had carefully noted mentally. Mum got him some cards to give to me. I looked at Alan with amazement, when I opened the one he had managed to sign himself. The effort that would have gone into signing that card said everything about what I meant to him.

How had he done it? That was when he explained to me how one of the carers had set him up in the kitchen, with the mobile arm support, so he could do it. This had been only days before he had stopped being able to use the support for feeding himself.

In the evening, after dinner we watched a video tape of an old Victor Borge show. Mum had brought it with her. It gave us what we needed more than anything else that day: it gave us a good laugh.

Running Out of Ammunition

Post Christmas 2005

Alan caught a cold. On the first morning of the cold he tried to stand up, but couldn't. He intended to walk the short distance from the bed to the glide-about chair, which he had been using since early December. His walking was much more awkward now, and I couldn't manage to walk him any further than a short distance, without help. The manual handling belt was necessary all the time, to keep him steady. But that morning, he was suddenly unable to stand. We were both shocked. It was so unexpected.

Much to my dismay, the immediate response of the company providing our care was to insist upon a hospital bed for him downstairs where we had the mobile hoist. We didn't have hoists upstairs to help get him in and out of our bed. It was the reason I had wanted the ceiling hoists so badly: I had seen this day coming. I had gone to a private company before Christmas and placed an order – fed-up with waiting for positive advice from the occupational therapist, on which I could act. The ceiling hoists were due to be installed very soon, but it wouldn't wait: 'health and safety rules.' Oh, how I grew to hate the words 'health and safety'!

They ordered the bed through the hospice. I wasn't given a choice, and nor was Alan, not if we wanted to keep our carers. Of course, I could do what I liked if I looked after Alan on my own, but I couldn't look after him on my own.

The bed came straight away. It was amazing how quickly something we didn't want was organised! Michael emptied all the furniture from the dining room – including the bloody dining room table – into the garage for me; so I could make the room into Alan's bedroom. I told myself that, at least, it meant he could still be cared for at home, but in the process, our life and our relationship was being eroded. So was our home. It started to feel as if we were living in a nursing home.

The next day Alan could stand again. I was over the moon. I hoped this would mean he could stay upstairs with me; that we would not be forced to use the hospital bed, for the moment. But the bed was in, and the care company would not agree to him going back upstairs. He never went upstairs again.

I cancelled the order for the ceiling hoists. There was no point now, but I knew that moving Alan downstairs like this was going to have a terrible effect on him, on us both.

My fears would prove to be correct: Alan's will to live was dealt a severe blow and began to slip away. It was the beginning of the end – sharing a bed was virtually all we had left of our relationship. Now that too was gone.

In reality, the hospital bed would have been installed at some point. Without it, Alan would have been trapped in the bedroom upstairs. Downstairs we had a shower room – finally! At least, if he was downstairs we could go out together, and I could attempt to give him some quality of life. But I am not sure Alan ever saw it that way, and I wish it could have been handled differently. Because others took charge without involving him, he was being treated like a child. He was not given the opportunity to be involved in the decision. Others decided what was best for him, including having to live. I think this made him angry. I think he was angry at me as well, even though I wasn't given a choice either. Up until the arrival of the hospital bed, he had been involved in decisions so that he could still feel in control. The reality was that the disease had brought us to this point, but it should have been discussed with him. It was my job to ensure he maintained some control over what happened to him, or at least to feel as though he did. This was the only dignity he had left. But on this occasion and many others, I failed.

I didn't sleep downstairs with Alan, not until his last weekend.

He slept well enough, which was fortunate, because not all people do who have MND. I was likely to sleep better in our bed upstairs, and I had the baby monitor if he should wake and need me. It seemed sensible for me to get a good night's sleep, so I would be fit to look after him the next day. If I had known how little time we had left, I might have arranged for some sort of temporary bed, even if I didn't always use it. I could have slept upstairs some nights; but, because I was always so tired, I didn't think to do it, and Alan never asked me to. I always felt guilty, leaving him on his own downstairs, but I couldn't share his hospital bed, in any case, and it was being able to feel the other's body and their warmth that was important.

So much for trying to maintain that 'normal' relationship everyone had talked about! No more listening to the radio in bed together, on a Sunday night; listening to David Jacobs playing the song from Mack and Mable: "I Won't Send Roses"– the song that has stayed in my memory from those times. No more drifting off to sleep with my head resting on his chest, reassured by the sound of his heart beating in steady rhythm along with mine.

So I was angry as well. We were completely frustrated in all our attempts to maintain some sort of normal life, and our home was being taken over in every sense. The only thing we hung on to was each other, and bit-by-bit, we were losing each other to the disease.

9 January 2006

I took Alan to the hospice. We had booked a respite week, and I was going away for a couple of days. I didn't really want to go. But everyone said I needed a proper break.

Because the hospital bed had been requested for our home, it was assumed Alan could no longer stand safely, or walk, and that he needed to be hoisted everywhere. But he could still stand and walk with aids; the hospice had not checked with us, or even with their own physiotherapist, who had seen Alan only the week before.

He wasn't put in the room he was expecting; the one he had been in on the previous two occasions. They usually tried to give people the same room, and I knew he would be happy, or as happy as he could be, with that room. It made it easier for me to leave him.

But they had arranged to put him in a different room: one with ceiling hoists. I didn't know, not until I carried his things in from the van. Alan was still in the van, oblivious for the moment. For health and safety reasons, the hospice had decided they could not allow him to stand or walk. I knew he would not be happy and I was upset for him.

I didn't want to leave him there, but I had booked to go away. I was torn over what to do. It was the first time, since he had been diagnosed, that I was going away on my own. It was difficult enough going somewhere and leaving him, let alone leaving him in this way.

I knew how important it was for him to keep on trying to stand and walk. On an emotional level it was important for him to try to maintain the muscles in his legs. Once the muscles weakened there was no getting them back. Physically, he liked to be able to stand and stretch his legs, and was happier having a pee in a standing position.

It was important for me as well. While he could stand, it was easier to look after him at home. It also made it easy for me to rub the backs of his legs and buttocks; something still to share a laugh over. He would go, 'Um, that's nice,' with a naughty chuckle. It was one of the few physical pleasures he got these days, although that wasn't the reason that I did it. You could say that it was a bonus. I did it to maintain the circulation and help prevent sores. These happen when someone stays sitting or lying in one position for too long. My mother had suggested it.

Standing there looking at that room with the hoists, I just wanted to take him home. I felt awful. Some respite!

A couple of weeks after he came home, Alan and I had a meeting with a senior member of the hospice staff. I didn't want to go through this again. It was hard enough for us both as it was, putting Alan in the hospice, without things like this happening. Of course, the hospice didn't want to put us through this either. We all realised there had been considerable misunderstanding and miscommunication over Alan's abilities. This had not been helped by the fact that they had not seen him in the day centre, not since before Christmas (almost a month). However, because we asked for the hospital bed they were obliged to make sure that they were meeting all health and safety regulations on their own premises, and lower than usual staffing levels that week compounded the problem.

We agreed to communicate more effectively with one another in future, and to make every effort not to repeat the episode. It was never repeated. The hospice staff only ever wanted to be helpful, and they did what they could in the last months of Alan's life.

There was little in the next three months that either of us would have been sad to miss. In fact, I wish our life together had been allowed to end then. I wish that the law would have allowed Alan the right to choose when to end his life – for him to have had the freedom and dignity of choice. Then I would have known that he had only lived for as long as he wanted to live and that he only suffered what he could stand to suffer. Not knowing whether his last days were unbearable is a torture that will never go away for me.

The last three to four months of Alan's life are mostly a blur, except for the things I would prefer to forget. They remain all too vivid. Only my diary and specific events have enabled me to place any kind of timing on what happened. From now on the over-riding feeling was one of total desperation, accompanied by anger and depression.

I tried to ensure that Alan could maintain some kind of control, in a situation in which neither of us had any real control. How did I ever expect to win? Somehow, I still kept battling on. I couldn't entertain the thought of not winning, although I don't know what winning meant, other than keeping Alan as comfortable and in control as I could. But I was running out of ammunition.

When grief took its hold, after Alan died, it was these last months that affected me most, and still remain uppermost in my mind. We were simply biding time, as best we could. Until this point, Alan said he felt he had some quality of life. I wanted my 'full of life' Alan back. I wanted the Alan who was always planning something – pushing me on. I expect he wanted his Nicola back, the one who would have to find something to worry about, because she didn't really have anything worth worrying about. But we both knew this would never be. Somehow, we just had to get each other through the remaining days.

Alan was thinking more and more about escaping; going to Switzerland to die.

I tried to make the best of things, aware that Alan was giving up; so I made Alan's 'bedroom' as comfortable and homely as possible. At least, from the bed he could look out at the garden. Although he didn't enjoy gardening, he did enjoy spending time in the garden, and we had spent some of our happiest times there - with each other and with family and friends.

Life was very limited now. We hung on to whatever we could. I still managed to walk him the short distance to the glide-about chair, when he got up in the mornings. We walked a little further when the physiotherapists were present. The carers would not walk him any longer. In fact, they were not keen for me to walk him, if they were with us. I knew what this meant to Alan, though I needed the reassurance of someone else around in case he fell. So we had another battle. Finally it was agreed. They would allow him to walk, when they were with us, if I was the one who walked with him, using the manual handling-belt to help him balance. It was up to us, but they were on hand if Alan fell.

Then a carer arrived one morning, who had not been briefed properly. She told me I wasn't allowed to walk him while she was there. I did not react well! When she left, I screamed and screamed in sheer frustration. I was upset and angry. No one seemed to understand! Unless we held on to what little we had, there wasn't any point in Alan living. Our efforts were continually being undermined.

From now on, the hours must have seemed endless for him. He had so much time to think. Other than watch television, or listen to the radio, that was all he could do on his own now – think. I was around for most of the time, but always doing, doing whatever needed to be done.

They say that when a person is nearing the end of their life, they reflect a lot on their past. Alan always said he had had a wonderful life.

Born in December, he was a Sagittarian. Apparently, for people of this sign, the journey is more important than the arrival. Whatever one's thoughts are about astrology, it fitted Alan well. It had been quite a journey from his birth at Lansdowne Gardens, South Lambert in London. He described himself as a cockney, although he didn't match the usual preconception of one. He did, however spend a large proportion of his youth within the sound of Bow Bells.

I am sure that the memories of his mother would have come back to him. Her name was Lillian. His father used to call her 'Lily' spelt 'like the flower'. She was a quiet, introverted person who found her boys a handful, especially Alan – he was the mischievous one, as he loved to tell me. He would recount with a mixture of glee and some remorse his childish pranks, and the fact that his poor mother had to chase him round the large parlour table in order to chastise him, with him shouting at her: 'You'll have to catch me first.'

That would have been in the flat at Tower Bridge. The flat was above the Westminster Bank, where Alan's father worked as a bank messenger. But during the war he was sent to work in factories, making engines for the war effort; first to Solihull and then to Slough. And this meant a lot of disruption for the family, as it had for so many other families during the war, but Alan was luckier than many; his family, though not wealthy, was close-knit and happy. Even when Alan's brother was separated from them, because he stayed on at the grammar school in Solihull, when the rest of the family moved back to the south, Alan and his brother kept in touch with each other through letters. Alan and his mother and father moved in with his father's sister, Aunt Lillian. She lived in Summer Road, East Molesey. From there, Alan's father cycled to Slough each day. It was easier than moving back to Tower Bridge, and avoided the bombing of central London. It also meant Alan spent a lot of his early years with his cousins, Rosie and Joan.

I wonder now, as he lay imprisoned by MND, unable to move, whether he remembered those joyous, youthful times when he never sat still. I know how happy he was at the house in Summer Road, because he took me there once and showed me the place by the river where he used to play. There was a small bridge and a pathway along the edge of the river-bank. He talked sometimes of his childhood holidays. They all used to go to Littlehampton, where they stayed in a small converted railway carriage – Alan, his brother, mother and father, aunt and cousins. There was that day when the usual seaside fun was augmented by Alan's adventurous nature: he succeeded in going missing while they were all on the beach. His frantic parents thought they had lost him to the River Arun, but he turned up an hour later, chirpy and oblivious to the panic he had caused.

Perhaps he thought about how his life could have taken a different path: of what might have been. He was obviously good at cycle racing, so perhaps he wondered what his life would have been like, had he been successful at this rather than in business. It may be that National Service got in the way of his passion, or that he accepted it as only a dream, but I hope that the many memories he must have had, of riding a bike at top speed, feeling the rush of the wind, while he pumped hard on the pedals with fit and active legs, helped to pass the leaden hours.

Many times now, when I think of the wonderful journeys we had, the incredible places we saw, and the people we met, our trips together playback through my mind, almost as though I am watching a film. I wonder whether it was like that for Alan. Did he, I wonder, remember riding the camel to the pyramids, the time we went to Cairo together, just as he had done when he visited them, at the end of his National Service? He had tried to persuade me to go on one, but I travelled separately on the tour bus. He was to try once more, when we went to Dubai; a ride into the desert to watch the sunset. I am sure that that ride would have stirred memories of the times, all those years before, when he had ridden with some friendly local Bedouin and taken photographs of life in the Egyptian desert; the ones I had found in the trunk in the garage. But he couldn't persuade me to get on a camel! It was just too far out of my comfort zone. Now though, I wish I had gone with him in Dubai. He might have told me some of those stories.

Was it his National Service posting that gave him his love of travel? Only a couple of years before being diagnosed, Alan went to Nepal. I didn't want to go, so he went alone. He would have liked me to go, but knew it was not for me. He remembered my reaction to the photographs he had taken when he was in India – so much poverty – having stopped off in Delhi, on the way back from a business trip to Japan, in the 1980s. He knew my limits after all the years we had been together. He also knew that I didn't want to spoil the trip for him. For him, the country had a magnetic pull. He had to go. He wanted to see Mount Everest and walk the streets of Kathmandu before he died. Somewhere, deep inside, there was a romantic side to him.

He phoned me soon after he arrived in Kathmandu. He couldn't wait to tell me that he had shared the first class aeroplane cabin with Prince Philip, who was also on his way to Nepal. He was going there to attend a conference for the World Wildlife Fund. Other than security people, Alan was the only person allowed to travel in the cabin. He thought I would be pleased to hear that all the checks on his character found him to be of no security risk to the Prince. It amused him that even a member of the Qatar royal family wasn't able to share the cabin, although it was probably because one prince was considered quite enough for the staff to look after.

The disease must have been especially unbearable for someone who had been so active, so in control of his life. He had needed these qualities, in order to achieve what he did in his business life. But for him getting a hole in one – which he did – gave him greater satisfaction than being successful in business; he always underestimated his business achievements. Yet he achieved a great deal. He had gone from a job as a Sales Executive for The Design Group in 1957, to being made Managing Director of that same company, by 1967. He had opened wholly-owned subsidiaries in Paris, Milan, Brussels and Stockholm, while holding that position. And, importantly, this had led eventually to setting up Parlour Wood with Ron. But, the journey was always more important than the arrival.

And that was what I think he enjoyed about his business life. Ron and Alan's clients had included Ford, Gillette, Hasbro, Nintendo, as well as many others. Alan did it because he found it exhilarating, but as a result he also contributed directly to other people's lives, not least the lives of the people who worked for him. He was generous- hearted, and always cared for the people he employed. He could and should have felt good about that.

I like to think that, in these hours, alone with only his thoughts, he was able to appreciate what he had achieved during his life. But he was a humble man, and I know he had a tendency to underestimate, not only his achievements, but also himself.

Nevertheless, as he was not the sort of person to dwell on disappointments, he would have tried to concentrate on all that had been good about his life. He must have prayed often that I would be able to do the same, and it is a great pity that we did not have the time to reminisce, even a little, together. But there was never time, once the disease began to take over our life.

To me, his life was all too short. I heard somewhere: 'A flame that burns twice as bright, burns half as long.' This would be a good description of Alan and his life. I am glad I picked that flame.

27 January 2006

We went to one of Alan's meetings for Pedigree Group. It helped to pull us up out of the doldrums. The meeting was held at a hotel near us, so I would not have far to drive. The directors tried to make it as easy as possible for me. We all had lunch together in the hotel lounge afterwards – just something light. Alan could still swallow and enjoy most foods, although he had gone off wine, as it irritated his throat, and caused him to choke. The whole day was just what we needed. It helped to make us feel happier and more positive than we had been able to feel in a long time – Alan still had something to offer. He was allowed to feel like a human being. And for me, it was good to see a little of my Alan still there.

We would never get over the hospital bed, but for the moment we managed not to let it affect us, not as much as it had at the beginning. Alan told me that he felt he still had some quality of life. I took this to mean that he still wanted to live, but perhaps he was just telling me he appreciated all that I was doing, that he knew how much I loved him.

Sometimes I found it hard to show him. There was so little time for affection. He had to make do with trying to see it in the way that I cared for him, and ignoring the frustration and anger I showed to the disease. I had to find affection in his words of support and the look in his eyes. Those eyes, those bright twinkling eyes, which attracted me at the very beginning, were still there. It was in these things that we still found each other. Somehow we still pulled the love through.

20 February 2006

We had a demonstration of the computer software that would help Alan communicate. It was the same software I described earlier, like that used by Stephen Hawking. The possibility that Alan would be able to speak to the end was unlikely, so I wanted us to be prepared, and have various options up our sleeves. For instance, one of the carers produced a communication book, which listed all the things Alan needed or asked for during a normal day – from the time he got up in the morning to the time he went to bed at night. It was intended that, if there was any uncertainty, we could point to something on the list, and he could signal, possibly by a wink, if it was what he wanted. But the software would be more like him speaking, so we had it to try for a month. I didn't realise how much effort would be required on my part to get him to spend any time with it. If he couldn't speak, he didn't want to live.

End February 2006

Alan decided to have the feeding tube. My fiftieth birthday was imminent, and looking back, I think it was my birthday that motivated him to go on living.

My fiftieth could not have been more different to my fortieth. For my fortieth we were in St Moritz, and I managed to end up with two celebrations as a result. Looking back, this was probably just as well.

On the day of my fortieth birthday, Alan took me for lunch at a chic restaurant, called La Marmite, located on one of St. Moritz's highest peaks. He had been along the previous day, to organise a table next to the window. The view from the restaurant is stunning, and from our table we could look straight out and down at the valley and lake. Virtually everything was white, apart from buildings and little skiers making their way down the piste. The snow glistened in the bright sunlight. We both had a glass of champagne. I ordered my favourite – truffles with pasta and olive oil – and I think Alan had the same, but I can't remember for sure. I do remember that we chose to eat lightly, because he had booked somewhere special for dinner that night.

My real birthday treat was delayed until May, when Alan took me to Tuscany. We stayed in two gorgeous hotels, one in Florence, and one overlooking the town of San Gimignano. I said at the time that I would like to go back for my fiftieth, and have lunch again at the vineyard that we went to in Montalcino. We bought a bottle of Brunello Di Montalcino Reserva 1990 to mark the occasion, and to keep for my fiftieth. Alan couldn't even enjoy this with me when we got to my fiftieth birthday, because of the way wine affected him.

We didn't have a big celebration planned for my fiftieth. In fact, all I wanted was one simple luxury. I hadn't had a lie-in for ages, probably not since before China. One of the carers had agreed to let herself in, at eight o'clock in the morning, so I could stay in bed. She was going to bring me a cup of tea. I hadn't had a cup of tea in bed since the early days of the stairlift. For me, this was the best birthday present I could receive, other than a miracle for Alan.

But Alan had some surprises planned for my landmark birthday!

The doorbell went. I thought my alarm clock had gone off, and then remembered that I hadn't set it. The doorbell went again. That's

odd I thought. The carer must have forgotten she should be letting herself in this morning. Then it went again. I looked at my bedside clock. It
was 7.15 am, not 8.00 am and the person at the door had resorted to the
doorknocker. Presumably they thought the bell didn't work.

Alan didn't call me. Usually he would. I expect he was hoping
the carer would finally remember and that I wouldn't have to get up.

Eventually I did and I wasn't happy. Fine start to my fiftieth! I
thundered down the stairs at 7.20 am and unbolted the door. I could see
a stranger on the other side through the glass in the door. He was holding something, but he was holding it down, so I couldn't see what it was.
I opened the door. I must have looked angry and then stunned. I just
stood there. He pushed the biggest bouquet of white flowers I had ever
seen towards me. He didn't look very happy, having spent twenty minutes trying to raise someone.

I didn't say thank you. I took the bouquet from him, and stared
into those flowers as though someone had just handed me a wreath for
Alan's coffin. I hate white flowers on their own; they mean funerals to
me.

I don't know if Alan asked for white flowers. He had never been
a person to buy me flowers. There had been only three occasions prior
to this that he had given me a bouquet of flowers: Valentine's Day, two
weeks earlier, once before Christmas, and the other time over twenty
years earlier when I returned from a sales conference in Barbados.

On that occasion my flight had been diverted to Frankfurt, owing
to mechanical problems. I had finally arrived back at Heathrow almost
a day later than scheduled. Alan came to meet me and presented me
with a beautiful bouquet of lemony yellow, orange, blue and red flowers
wrapped in orange tissue and cellophane. I can picture them now. He
looked so pleased to see me, and I was so glad he had made time to
come from work to fetch me. He threw his arms around me and we

hugged each other as though we had not seen each other in years. I felt the warmth of his love and I felt safe. Vibrant coloured flowers always reminded me of this special moment.

In a way, it was because Alan had rarely bought me flowers that he didn't know what kind of flowers I liked, and this was adding to my escalating feelings of anger. I don't particularly like big bouquets either. It meant having to find enough vases, and then rearranging them all into the vases. It just wasn't my thing, and these days even less so. I would never be able to get this bouquet into a single vase!

Alan had just wanted to make my day – with a beautiful bouquet of flowers. It was one of the few options open to him to organise a surprise for me; even then he had needed the help of a carer. It had simply all gone wrong. At any other time in my life I would have taken it in my stride and accepted them gracefully, as a lovely thought. I had on Valentine's Day, when he organised a slightly smaller bouquet of blue and purple flowers. I don't care much for purple either. Nevertheless, I was pleased with the thought. Then, the thought had been enough, but not today. And I never thought to ask him later if he had ordered white flowers, or whether that's what the florist had decided to do. I never thought to ask, because I was thinking that had he bought me flowers more often, he would have known my favourite colours – the yellows, oranges and reds of the flowers he had given me on my return from Barbados.

It didn't occur to me that he didn't want any of this to happen. I just assumed it was his fault. He knew how important the lie-in and cup of tea in bed were to me. Why did he have to spoil it by ordering flowers – white flowers! White flowers delivered at 7.00am!

So he had to bear the brunt, and watch me raving like a lunatic at him. I tore up the flowers and I threw them out of the conservatory doorway into the garden. Alan was crying – I left him crying as I ran upstairs, leaving him alone until the carer turned up. I was so cross. I couldn't be sympathetic to his tears. I couldn't see it from his point of view. He wanted that day to be special, but everything was beyond his control. If only the disease hadn't taken away the use of his arms, he could have given me a cuddle and it would all have been alright.

And the agony didn't stop at the flowers. Alan had also booked, with the carers help, a restaurant for lunch. It was one that he knew I liked. In fact, I had asked to go there, which is why he told me that it had changed since we last went. The restaurant advised this when the carer made the booking for Alan. Why hadn't I listened? Why hadn't I phoned to check? But I organised everything these days. I didn't want to be involved in organising my own birthday treat.

After what had happened with the flowers, he must have been worrying about it. Michael came over during the morning. He had agreed to have lunch with us and do all the driving. When we got to the restaurant, Alan suggested we leave him in the van in order to check it out before we took him in.

'If it's not alright,' he said 'we can go somewhere else.' It wasn't alright, and it could not have been more different to Jöhri's Talvo, the restaurant in Champfèr, near St Moritz, to which Alan had taken me for dinner, on the day of my fortieth birthday. That restaurant had been warm, cosy and romantic and the food was fabulous. This restaurant, however, was more suited to a child's party, especially as the menu consisted of things like hamburgers and chips. But by now, I was past caring. I just couldn't face the thought of trying to find somewhere else at this late stage. It was easier to stay and have lunch there, and I felt it was partly my own fault. I had devolved the responsibility to Alan and his carers. It was unfair of me to expect too much.

But I should have gone back to the van and told him, so we could go somewhere else. When I pushed him up to the table he was looking around and in tears. I put my hand on his and said, 'It's OK.' We both knew it wasn't.

The events of that day marked a turning point for both of us. The disease was just proving too much for us both.

When we arrived home from the restaurant, he needed to get to the bathroom quickly. I found myself standing there in the bathroom with his son, and just crying and saying: 'I hate this disease.' I was probably voicing Alan's feelings as well. He didn't say anything. He didn't have to, because I had said it. His son put his arms around me, as Alan would have wanted to do – as I needed Alan to do.

If Alan had any desire to go on living for any length of time after my fiftieth birthday, it must have completely left him on that day. If he had any doubts about wanting to die, the events of that day probably dispelled them, and my obvious disappointment had been the final trigger. It had been important to me that I should have happy memories of this day. It was not only my fiftieth; it was likely to be my last birthday with Alan, and it had been spoiled. I couldn't suppress my disappointment – on my birthday, we had both been cheated by the disease again.

The day after my birthday, with me at the end of my tether, Alan was taken into the hospice.

9 March 2006

I was visited by a back-care specialist. She had been recommended by Alan's physiotherapist from the hospice, who thought I would benefit from some professional advice – to protect my back. Although the recommendation had been made before Christmas, I had not been able to get in contact with the specialist until January, because of everything else which had been going on, and this turned out to be the first available appointment.

The lady who came was kind, professional in her approach, and clearly very experienced. I had thought she would give me the sort of advice that I had had from my osteopath, but soon realised that she offered much more than this. I realised I would have benefited enormously from an earlier visit. She was very aware of the difficulties we were facing. She was not surprised that things had got on top of me. In fact, she was horrified when she saw the way in which I had been left to cope. She couldn't understand how I had managed for as long as I had and most particularly, why Alan had not been entitled to continuing care at the last assessment. She was extremely knowledgeable about the help available.

She asked me a lot of questions, including things like how tall Alan was – a lot taller than me. She asked me how much he weighed – almost one and half times my weight. Well that had been his weight the last time we had been able to weigh him. But we had been making every effort to maintain his weight. We understood that this, together with the exercises, would help maintain his muscles, and therefore help to slow the effect of the disease.

All these things were important for Alan's sake, but had taken their toll on me. It was obvious to her that I was physically exhausted, and that I needed not only more people support, but also the right equipment. The equipment we had at the time was the dreaded hospital bed, a mobile hoist that was not meant to be used by one person alone, a glide-about chair and a shower chair. The latter had become very uncomfortable for Alan, and was inappropriate for his needs. The correct shower chair should have been available via our social services, but no one had told me. Not until this person did.

When I was on my own and needing to move Alan, it was easier for me to get him to stand, and quickly push the glide-about chair under him, rather than use the mobile hoist to transfer him. I was alone with Alan for most of the day. If Alan fell while I was doing this, I would have to call the ambulance services. That was what I had been told to do, except that when I had used this service, the ambulance staff who came said they were not allowed to help me get Alan up. Health and safety rules! They did help. But when I told the back care specialist, she told me they should not have said this. It was not correct. I could call an ambulance. But in the meantime I had been left fearing a fall. What was I supposed to do? Misinformation!

Following this visit, the hospice completed the paperwork for another assessment for continuing care. A senior member of staff at the hospice had also been surprised when I told her that we did not have continuing care. The specialist and the hospice staff worked together. They coordinated with one another to make the case on our behalf. Coordination: that was a first! On top of this, the back-care specialist contacted social services to sort out more suitable equipment. She knew exactly what support Alan was entitled to, and who to contact to make it happen, and she pursued it all for me. She was a gift from heaven! If only I had seen her earlier, what a difference she could have made to our lives in those last few months!

The occupational therapist came from social services. She agreed that I needed ceiling hoists. It was March, and I had been trying to get someone to give advice since last October. That was why I had ordered some myself. But when Alan had to move downstairs, I only managed to cancel the order, not to get someone to come back to tell me what I could do downstairs.

Finally, social services said they would get a technician to come and measure up for a hoist above Alan's bed and another above his chair in the lounge. I was looking forward to reclaiming some of our home. To use the mobile hoist, it had been necessary to move still more furniture into the garage, and push all the chairs back to the wall, to create enough space to allow the mobile hoist to be manoeuvred into position, when we needed to use it. The prospect of making the sitting room look less like an institution was already making me feel better. We had been living under occupation, but at last we were being allowed to reclaim some ground.

There is a pattern to the form of MND that Alan had. A case-worker, with the correct training, should be able to spot the stages and know what, when and how to bring in the resources required. This had not happened. It only started to happen after the back care specialist became involved, but by then it was too late.

13 March 2006

Alan went into hospital to have the feeding tube fitted. He went straight from the hospice to the hospital.

On the day Alan had to go to hospital, I went to the hospice, to make sure everything he needed went with him, and I didn't want him to be alone when he got to the hospital. He could talk, but it was a tremendous effort for him. He went by ambulance, and I followed in the van.

Alan was put in a room on his own, and again he had his own bathroom. This was very nice, except that the room was a long way from the nurses' station. What was he supposed to do, when he needed something? He couldn't push the alarm button. He couldn't use his hands! Nor could he shout loud enough. His voice was very weak.

The whole business of him going into hospital for the feeding tube, had been on my mind for some time, partly because we had been given so little information, and partly because it was something else we would need to adapt to. We only knew what we had been told at the Royal Brompton Hospital, before Christmas.

The local hospital which was fitting the feeding tube, had provided virtually no information. We had been sent a letter with the date and time, and very little more. We learnt when Alan was admitted, that he would have to swallow an endoscope under local anaesthetic.* This was the first time it had been mentioned. They would not be able to give him a general anaesthetic because no anaesthetist was available; not without re-booking for another time. Alan was terrified because of his difficulty swallowing. He had been through a similar experience, for an investigative procedure, over a year before – the one that had led to the diagnosis that he had IBS. Then the local anaesthetic had not worked and the consultant had to abort and use an alternative test. That was before Alan was experiencing the level of difficulties with swallowing which he had now.

Alan agreed to go ahead, largely because the hospice doctor visited him later in the day. I was anticipating, when I left him, that we might have to cancel, get Alan home and re-book. The hospice doctor managed to speak to the hospital staff, and together they persuaded Alan that everything would be alright. By the time I went back in the evening, Alan was happier. Furthermore, he had been moved to a room by the nurses' station, again due to the intervention of the doctor from the hospice. I felt relieved and appreciated the care the hospice was giving. I didn't feel quite so alone. Someone else was fighting for Alan.

It was fortunate the operation went ahead. A delay would have caused Alan very real distress in the weeks to come.

All the time he was in hospital, I worried about him. So when I went to visit him just after the feeding tube had been put in, and heard him call several times for a bedpan, I flipped. I flipped easily these days. I could hear him while I was walking along the corridor to his room. Hearing him having to call more than once, distressed me so much that I found myself shouting at the staff at the nurses' station, 'If he shits the bed, it's your fault.' I know this sounds dreadful, but I didn't care what anyone thought of me. All I cared about was Alan, and how degrading he would find it, if they didn't reach him with a bedpan, in time. I was angry. Going into hospital for the feeding tube had been a difficult decision. Alan didn't want to prolong his life through it; he simply wanted to minimise his own suffering. I was furious. The very system that would not help him to die, would not look after him properly or with dignity.

He had always been concerned about losing control, and making a mess in the bed, or anywhere. I felt responsible because I had left him to fend for himself, and he wasn't able to do so. I felt guilty. I even questioned my feelings for him. Did I still love him? How could I do this to him? It was the only time I didn't stay with him in hospital. I simply couldn't do it, even though I knew how difficult it would be for him, without my help. How could I abandon him, when he so clearly needed me? If I still loved him, surely I would have found the strength to stay with him. I wish I could have been strong enough to stay with him, as I had always done before. I was angry with the staff. However, I was even angrier with myself.

He told me as the nurses came in with the bedpan, that he hadn't been calling for long. I calmed down with Alan's words, and helped the nursing staff. They were very kind and understanding about my outburst. There appeared to be only three or four nurses trying to look after a massive ward with individual rooms for each patient. For other patients, without Alan's disabilities the rooms would have been perfect. But such an environment did not make it easy for them to look after him, although I know he would have appreciated the privacy it gave him.

The next shock was seeing the feeding tube in him, for the first time. It wasn't what I had expected at all. The tube itself was very long – nothing like the ones we had been shown at the Royal Brompton Hospital. It was wider as well, apparently so it would be less likely to get blocked. We would have to curl it round several times and tape it down, to stop it catching on clothing or getting in the way. It was a shock, and we were stuck with it, just like everything else with the disease. Now I had to learn how to feed him via the tube, and I would be doing this much sooner than we had anticipated; his condition deteriorated rapidly from this moment.

Alan returned to the hospice for a week, to try to give me a longer rest. I didn't ask him, because I didn't think I could cope at home. He needed much more support than I could give. Regardless of the fact that I was still exhausted, I simply did not have suitable support in place at home.

This was one of the worst times in the whole disease. I wanted to care for Alan at home, but I didn't know how I was going to do it. On top of this, I had promised him we would be in this together, so I felt I was letting him down. My heart was being torn into shreds.

15 March 2006

Alan came home from the hospice. Although he had been away for three weeks, I did not feel rested. During the last few days, I had been backwards and forwards to the hospital and hospice. I couldn't leave Alan without my support. He had been through so much, and I missed him.

On the day he came home, I was frantic about how I would manage. I had started to think about live-in care, but had yet to find time to look into it. I didn't want it and I didn't think Alan would either. It would be very intrusive, but how else would I cope? In an effort to start talking about it, I told Alan that we might have to consider a nursing home. I wasn't convinced I could get the level of support I needed at home quickly enough. I wish I had never said it. He wasn't interested. He just wanted to die, and I just felt as though I was letting him down. It wasn't what I wanted, but I had never expected to be so alone in trying to make life bearable until he died.

The Macmillan Nurse came to see us that day and Alan announced, in front of her, that he wanted to die. He had lost control of virtually every aspect of his life. This was the first time he had said it since early January, but this time I knew he meant it. I felt that what I had said made him feel this way. I had been forced to consider something I didn't want any more than he did, but how can I be sure he knew that? I felt as though I was abandoning him when he needed me most, and I felt terrible. I had lost him long ago to the disease. He didn't want pity. He had had a good life. He didn't want to go into a nursing home. In fact he didn't want to be looked after at all; to be totally reliant on others. He had said that when he was diagnosed. He just wanted to be allowed to die when he had had enough. It was his life after all, and yet he wasn't even allowed control over whether he wanted it to end.

And I didn't want to be in the position I was, before he went into the hospice –reduced to shouting at him over something that was beyond his control and making it even worse for him.

Within a couple of days I was doing exactly that; I was woken in the middle of the night by him calling to me. I walked out onto the landing, and as I did so, I heard him say, 'There's a burglar in the house.' I was scared out of my wits. I crept downstairs and checked the front door. It was still locked, and there was no sign of a break-in anywhere in the house.

I reacted a bit like a mother who has just pulled her child back before it runs in front of a passing car. I felt a mixture of fear and anger. The mother is scared because the child nearly got killed. She is angry because the child didn't stop and think first.

If there had been an intruder, Alan could have put me in a dangerous position. Surely, it would have been safer to have left me in bed? I flew into a rage, and told him what I thought of being got out of bed. I overreacted, but I was very tired. It upset him so much that he started to sob. He thought the disease had made me hate him. This was the sec-

193

ond time I had reacted this way, if I exclude the chocolate pudding incident, which had been quite minor by comparison. As soon as he said 'You look as though you hate me,' I stopped shouting. Imagine how I felt, that I had made him feel this way. It was the last thing I wanted to do. What he had seen was fear not hate. But I was too tired to explain. I didn't really understand myself. I didn't want to be shouting and screaming at him. It was a release; but in the process I had upset him. It was the last thing I wanted to do.

I hated the disease for what it was doing to Alan and to me. I was angry that it had left us both vulnerable. It prevented him from being my Alan, the Alan who would have been able to protect us. I was shouting at the disease. I did hate the disease, but not Alan. I was angry and scared.

It didn't occur to me, until later, that he must have had a bad dream. Why did he have to have this dream? Why? If he hadn't, and if I hadn't been so tired, and if we had been upstairs in our bed together, it would never have happened. So many 'ifs'! The effect was not positive. It left me feeling guilty that I had not been sympathetic. Lying there alone in the darkness, unable to move; he was scared too.

20 March 2006

We were again assessed for continuing care, and it was awarded.

But it was too late. I am sure the emotional effect on us both would not have been as great, had we received the right support earlier. Without someone to look after him, Alan would have died. The NHS finally recognised that his care was not simply personal care; it was a health need. He was totally reliant on others, like a baby. The medical profession could not help him to die, but until now the NHS had not been prepared to give us the help he deserved to go on living; it seemed inhuman.

Continuing care did not pay for everything, but it made a significant contribution. Importantly, we were now informed about available additional help. Why did it have to take so long! Why did I have to get so very close to the end of my tether? We were able to access more support during the day, in order to help me in the hours between the carers leaving, after getting Alan up in the morning, and returning to put him to bed at night.

Before this extra assistance was granted, I would dread Alan needing to go to the toilet. It was 'Sod's Law' that, when all help had walked out through the door, and I was on my own looking after him, he would need to go. It was probably because he was just as anxious as me.

We were also put in touch with Crossroads, an organisation that supports carers at home. This organisation, with its own carers, was able to give far more support than we had previously been led to believe. When I was first advised of the organisation, I was told that their resources were under considerable pressure. They were very stretched, like everyone else. On top of this, I was given the impression that they would not be able to provide personal care, such as help to the toilet if necessary. As a result, I had not pursued it before. But now we learned that, given the nature of MND, and its effect on the main carer, we would be considered a priority, and the carers were able to assist in personal care. As a result, I had the help of a Crossroads carer support worker for a few hours during the Saturday and Sunday of the last two weekends of Alan's life.

At last, the support seemed to be falling into place, although we were still waiting for the shower chair, and for ceiling hoists to be fitted. Now that Alan had been accepted for continuing care, all the papers for these aids had to be passed from the social services to the NHS – two different budgets! He died before either were fitted. I am not sure that they were ever ordered.

Had we been offered and received this support six months earlier, the quality of Alan's last months would have been better and much less fraught. It would have made a difference. It would have made a difference to the end of his life, and to the way I would feel after he died.

He didn't only have to deal with the impact of the disease on himself. Alan had to watch me crumbling under the pressure that the demands of the disease placed on us. He had to look on, helpless. It was torture. Yet he was amazing, and I told him so. I told him many times, because he was. The way he remained so calm, the way he used to come home and tell me about the people he met at the hospice; those also suffering from disabling terminal illnesses. He always compared his situation to theirs, and considered himself fortunate that he had been allowed a wonderful life before the disease. And through it all, he never lost his sense of humour.

But we were really losing the battle now. I had been able to continue standing and walking Alan, until the feeding tube was fitted. We had not realised that it would prevent him from walking altogether. It did, because we could not risk him falling and the tube becoming detached.

For some time, he had been using a solid box at the bottom of his bed to push against with his feet. This allowed him to push himself back up the bed if he slipped down. He also used it as a way of exercising his legs. The box was a bath step we had bought for getting in and out of the bath, which had become redundant before he had ever used it. Once he had the feeding tube this became the only means, other than physiotherapy, for him to exercise his legs. I would still stand Alan, from time to time, even after the feeding tube was fitted, if only to rub the backs of his legs and buttocks, to keep the circulation going.

But I will never forget the day he told me, 'I think the muscles in my legs are going.' My heart sank. I had noticed, but didn't want to say.

I knew what this meant to my racing cyclist!

At this stage in his life, I am certain that Alan simply wanted to be able to see me happy, and show me how much he loved me. Watching him slowly being taken from me in this way, how could I be happy? It was hopeless.

First week of April 2006

Alan became quite sick. The doctor gave him antibiotics, thinking he had a chest infection, but they didn't work. We tried one antibiotic after another without success.

But Alan had simply had enough. I discussed going to Switzerland with my mother. She said she would come with us to give me support.

In the meantime, we tried to live from day to day, planning wherever we could. Between the feeding tube being fitted, and Alan's last weekend, we did manage to go to another Pedigree board meeting together. We also managed to go out, with the help of my mother and a carer, on the Saturdays. Alan still found ways to make me laugh. Around that time there was a television production of Bleak House by Charles Dickens. Alan took to saying 'Shake me up, Judy', when we put him into the wheelchair, mimicking the wheelchair-bound character, Mr Smallweed.

Saturday, Easter weekend 2006

We all went to Kew Gardens. It was a massive effort, not least for Alan. But he wanted to go. The carer that day, who was from South Africa, had never been before. Alan liked the idea of taking her, still wanting to help others experience as much of life as possible. To the end he tried to make the best of life, even though he had made it clear he wanted to die. She was so excited about being at Kew, she telephoned her mother in South Africa, just to tell her where she was.

But Alan wasn't at all well. I was seeing the last of that wonderful sparkle in his eyes. Like the last burst of beautiful lemon flowers on the rhododendron tree in Cornwall, I would never see that sparkle again.

Easter Monday 2006

I didn't give Alan his vitamins and supplements. He was finding it harder and harder to swallow them without choking, and he was so unwell. It seemed cruel to go on giving them to him. Why had I been giving them to him for so long? Was it for him, or was it for me? However, he had taken them willingly every day. That morning I said to him, 'I can't see the point any more.' Was I letting go? Was I giving up on him, or was I simply accepting his need to die? I couldn't tell you; I don't know. I just wanted the disease to end for both of us, and I am sure he felt the same. The only problem was, I would survive the disease; he couldn't. We would both be rid of the disease, but I had to lose the person I loved more than anything in the process.

I think it was either that night, or possibly the next night, that I couldn't get his pillows comfortable, before I went to bed. It was so important to get them exactly right, so he could sleep. He had never disturbed me in the night, apart from that night when he thought there was a burglar in the house. And after my reaction to that incident, I expect he would have had to have been very uncomfortable to do so! I still felt awful about it. I always will.

I kept pulling him forward to adjust his pillows. They had to be in the right position to support his back, neck and head. He was a dead weight. The carers had left only a short while before. They usually made sure the pillows were right, before they went. But that night they didn't. It wasn't their fault. Alan just wasn't comfortable. It didn't matter how many times I pulled him forward and adjusted them, they still weren't right. I got quite cross. My arms were getting more and more tired and started to ache. My whole body ached, and I became more frustrated with each failed attempt to get him comfortable. I got more cross. I was cross with myself really, but when he became upset I thought, 'I've done it again. He thinks I hate him.' He wasn't being difficult. He just wasn't comfortable. It wasn't his fault, but I felt completely exasperated. Eventually, I just sat down on the floor beside his bed, with my back against the wall and cried. He was crying too. I felt awful, but I couldn't do anything. I so wanted him to be comfortable, but I couldn't make him so, no matter what I did. The disease was winning; I was losing.

That was when he said, 'You know my trunk has gone?' The muscles supporting his back had given up, and that was why he was having difficulty. I thought he was confirming his desire to go to Switzerland. He had always said 'When my trunk goes, that's it. I'll be off to Switzerland.' But perhaps he was trying to tell me he was dying. He was trying to warn me. If he was, I was in denial. I just didn't see it. We had been fighting for so long.

For more than twenty-five years he had been there to take care of me. He still wanted to. All he had ever typed into the computer which we had on trial, the one which could eventually help with communication, was 'I love you.' He saved the phrase and never typed anything else. It had been hard work for him to type just that short phrase. He used the pad behind his head to input each letter and his neck muscles had virtually gone. The effort must have been very great. But he wanted me to know he still cared for me, and he used any way he could to let me know. That was all he wanted to do while he was alive.

However, at some point my protector wouldn't be there any more. I would be on my own. He had been with me for more than a third of his life, but I had lived more of my life with him than without him. I didn't know anything else. I didn't want to. Life without him was unimaginable. I was in denial.

I wish that in that week before he died, I could have found the words to tell him how happy he had made me, before the disease took hold. I know he wanted to see me happy after that. He told me, 'You will have a wonderful life.' He said it as though he expected it of me. After all, life is for living. That was his attitude. That's why we both went China. But what he had now wasn't life – not for him. We both tried to make the disease easier on the other. But being happy, after China, was as impossible as finding the words turned out to be. All I managed was, 'It has been a wonderful life. But this bit has been so hard.' I don't know how he interpreted this. I didn't know what else to say and I didn't get the opportunity to elaborate. I was not expecting him to die so soon.

Yes, in these latter stages of the disease, when I woke up in the morning, I hoped I would find he had been allowed to die in his sleep. I had prayed for this, virtually since the hospital bed. Furthermore, whenever I went out in the last few weeks of his life, I would dread coming home; I would sit in the car, on the driveway, trying to summon the energy to go into the house. I was still being torn. I didn't want to live with the disease any more than he did, and I didn't want to lose him. I wanted my Alan back. That's what I said to him, 'I want my Alan back.' The pain in my heart was excruciating. I was pleading with him. 'I want my Alan back, and that can never be.' It must have been as painful for him to hear me as for me to say. He couldn't even put his arms around me. But I wasn't expecting him to die. I was in denial.

20 April 2006

We went to the Royal Brompton Hospital, for his second sleep test. He wasn't really well enough, but I didn't want to cancel, in case he needed to use the NPPV machine. His breathing was becoming very difficult. He needed to try different masks, because he had not got on well with what we had been given before Christmas, and I wanted to make sure I knew what to do, if his breathing became distressed. I was still trying to pre-empt anything that would make Alan uncomfortable, and make sure we could deal with it.

If I had known he would die a few days later, I would not have gone, especially as they didn't send the right ambulance to pick us up. It was a taxi ambulance, and Alan's wheelchair had to be upright for the whole forty-five minute journey into London. Even when I realised how we would have to get to the hospital, I still didn't want to cancel and re-book the sleep test, because Alan's breathing was deteriorating.

The journey was so uncomfortable for him. I held his hand tightly all the way. I didn't know what else to do.

It was a one-night stay and I stayed with him. I couldn't leave him, not after the last time with the feeding tube. I hadn't forgiven myself. And speech was getting very difficult for him. I usually understood what he needed or wanted, even if others didn't; so it helped if I was there to explain for him.

That night, as I lay beside him on the put-you-up, he said 'Together at last.' I think he wanted me to feel the magic he felt. But I didn't get it then. I was too exhausted from the effects of him being unwell, from the effort of getting him to the hospital. I was full of sorrow about everything.

Yet, this was our first night together in the same room, since that awful hospital bed had entered our life. I wish I had felt it. But I didn't. I replied, 'I love you. Good night, darling. Sleep tight.' I was thinking, please God let him sleep well, so I can get some sleep.

Alan improved while we were there. His sleep test went well! His oxygen levels were still good. We came away with a couple of different masks that he found more comfortable to use.

But, as soon as we got home, he started to deteriorate. I believe now that he had somehow managed to hang on. He wanted to get home.

I phoned the doctor who told me that it was possible Alan had a virus. This would explain why the antibiotics weren't working. However, he suggested we try one more course. I responded by telling him, 'I don't think it is a virus or an infection. I think it's the disease, and his system is shutting down.' Nevertheless, I got another prescription.

I felt he was giving up. In some ways, I was expecting him to die. However, because his oxygen levels were good, I was not expecting him to die within the next few days. In fact, I thought he could still go on for quite a while longer – months even. I was still thinking we would have to go to Switzerland.

Till All Our Fight be Fought

Saturday, 22 April 2006

It was the last weekend of the month. The winter had been long, and the spring colder than I ever remembered before. All the spring flowers were late.

'I don't feel like having a shower,' Alan managed to force out the words. But, Alan always feels like having a shower, I thought to myself. The only time he didn't have one was when he had to have bed baths in hospital. But, that morning, he asked for a bed bath.

Over the last two days in hospital, he had been lugged about quite a bit. At one point, there must have been five nurses in the room, getting him in and out of the hoist, in order to move him to and from the bed. Alan handled the disease with great courage, and hardly complained at all. Once, when I had been screaming with frustration, he said: 'I too feel like screaming sometimes.' He said it in a way that told me he understood. But he hardly complained at all, even though he never wanted to be looked after, to be totally dependent on others for everything. He rarely showed his frustration. Perhaps he let me do it for him.

Watching them move him, it might just as well have been me in that sling. I knew exactly what he was feeling.

He was being hauled about like a lump of meat in an abattoir. What respect for human life was this? There wasn't any dignity in it; none whatsoever. This was not respect for human life. His face looked blank. Yet, in his eyes, I could see how much he hated it. He said nothing, but I could see it. And still no one could help him to die.

The person in that hospital, and here with me now at home, was not my Alan. My Alan was that person who looked after me, who made decisions, who was always active and wanting to live life to the full. The face that looked at me now was blank.

That morning, I could see he didn't care, and the effort of getting to the shower was too much. He did not feel well. He had absolutely had enough.

My mother came over as usual, and I had a carer to help. A second carer, from Crossroads, came to help in the afternoon, with the idea that Mum and I could go out. But we weren't going anywhere; I didn't want to leave Alan, so we thought we would spend some time in the garden.

I had bought some geraniums, while I was at work the previous Tuesday. I wanted the garden to look especially beautiful for the summer, so Alan and I would have something we could still enjoy together.

When we went out into the garden, I noticed a long cluster of buds waiting to bloom on the wisteria which I had planted a few years before, because Alan liked wisteria. We both did. There was already one on the back wall of the house, and that one had lilac/blue flowers. Alan had been carefully training it into a lovely shape. Although he was not keen on gardening, he took great pride in this job, and had been doing it ever since we planted it the year after we moved into the house. I was training the second one over an arch which we had built together. This would be its first flowering, so I was particularly looking forward to it coming out and showing it to Alan. When it did come out, each flower on the bloom was white and fragrant. Though white, it was not the cold snow-white of the flowers in that ill-fated bouquet; it was white, warmed by a touch of pink. But he didn't get to see them.

It was a gloriously sunny day. We seemed to have missed out on the spring altogether, and gone straight from winter to summer. Alan said he would like to come outside with us. This was very unusual. But I was so pleased. I thought it meant he was feeling a bit better. On reflection, I should have realised. He knew how much I loved the garden; he knew this was the last time he would see me there – happy in the garden. That was how he wanted to see me – happy. The disease had made me so unhappy. But in the garden I was different. He would see his Nicola again, before he died.

We wheeled him into some shade, and I potted up the geraniums beside him. I wanted to be close to him. I don't know why. I just felt it was important to be near him. The carers came out as well, and helped in the garden. It was a happy scene, with lots of activity in the bright sunlight.

Alan sat in his wheelchair and watched. But his expression was blank. I suppose he was just taking it all in, and trying to hold onto the picture. After an hour or so, he said he wanted to go back in. He was getting uncomfortable. For a few months, he had been wearing a hyoscine patch* behind his ear, to reduce the saliva secretions in his throat. Until now, he could clear them from his throat, but since the morning he had been finding it difficult. This seemed to be affecting his breathing and adding to his discomfort. I said, 'Let me just finish this. Then we'll all go inside, and get you comfortable.' He waited patiently for the few moments I needed. But his expression remained blank.

When we went back in, he said he wanted to lie down on the bed. I think he thought that if his head was back he would be able to breathe more easily. We hoisted him onto the bed, but he still wasn't comfortable. So, after a while, we hoisted him into his riser/recliner chair. He still couldn't get comfortable. He tried the NPPV machine, but it didn't have the desired effect for him. We tried the bed again.

There he stayed until the carers came in the evening. He didn't want anything to eat. He hadn't the previous evening either. Alan had still been able to enjoy soft food, mainly meals made with pasta, up to a couple of weeks before. But the increasing incidence of choking distressed him, so he asked for his food to be liquidised. He was afraid of small pieces getting stuck in his throat. I had been shown how to help, and we had been able to control it. But nevertheless, it worried him. The first night that we had relied completely on the feeding tube was the night before, when we got back from the Royal Brompton Hospital. He just didn't have the energy to eat.

Before bedtime, after the carers went, he said to me: 'I'm tired. I want to die.'

'I know darling,' I replied gently. I was holding back the tears. I knew the disease had become totally unbearable for him. 'I have asked Mum if she would come with us to Switzerland. She said she would.' She wanted to be there to give me support, and I felt it would make it easier for Alan if he knew this; but I went on 'I would rather we didn't have to go, because of the thought of you being lugged around in ambulances, and air ambulances, and dying in another country. I really wish you could be allowed to die at home.' As I looked into his face, I knew we wanted the same and we were both so battle-weary. But we still didn't want to lose each other. The disease had brought us to this.

I went to bed, but I could hear him struggling to breathe over the baby monitor, so I went downstairs, to lie on the sofa near him. Neither of us could sleep. It was a long night.

For a while, he had been saying 'Ello' because he couldn't say 'Hello,' when I opened his curtains in the morning. He always had such a lovely smile on his face, as he said it. His eyes sparkled and he looked so pleased to see me. 'Good morning' had long gone. It was too much of an effort.

Sunday morning was no different, except that 'Ello' was barely audible.

My mother had tried to warn me that she thought Alan was dying. In a way I could see it, but part of me said there was a possibility he could go on living. I was being torn between so many conflicting thoughts. For his sake I hoped his suffering would end, but that would mean I would be left alone, without him. Part of me wanted him to go on living.

Alan's condition was much the same throughout the day. Death was close, but I didn't see it coming. It's just a virus, I thought – he'll get over it. His breathing had been fine at the hospital.

But he wasn't fine. The circulation in his legs was going. His breathing had become more distressed, largely because he couldn't clear the secretions from his throat, although I didn't realise this. I didn't call the doctor until Monday morning, because I didn't realise anything could be done, and I didn't want a duty doctor to come. Not knowing the background, a duty doctor might insist Alan went into hospital. Well, that was my fear, and I didn't want to risk it.

On the Monday morning, I asked Alan, 'Do you want me to call the doctor?' I was still trying to give him control of his life in whatever way I could. It was up to him. I needed to know what he wanted me to do. Over the weekend, we had started to resort to one wink for 'Yes'. If he didn't wink, it meant 'No'. Because there was so little volume in his voice, it was difficult to be certain of what he was saying. Winking helped to clarify his responses. He replied, 'Yes.' It was a whisper, but I didn't need any clarification. I heard him.

I asked him: 'do you want any treatment?' I have no idea what I meant by this. I don't think he did either. He looked at me blankly. So I said, 'Do you want to just be kept out of distress?'

'I am in distress.' Again, although faint, I heard his answer. He was in distress! I was distraught.

The disease was jeering at me 'Now I've got you. Now what are you going to do?' I called the doctor, but felt completely defenceless. When he came I repeated the question. I wanted the doctor to be left in no doubt that Alan didn't want to be kept alive. He wanted to be made comfortable. I was almost hysterical, as I asked the doctor to do whatever he could to make sure Alan would not be in any further distress. I couldn't bear seeing him in this state.

The Macmillan Nurse came from the hospice. Alan was due to go in for a respite week the following day. We didn't know what to do. If Alan was going to die, I wanted it to be at home. But, if he didn't die, I needed the rest to be able to look after him. We agreed to review it the next day.

I called Michael, and let him know that I thought his father was dying. Although I was saying the words, the words were not real. It was still unimaginable to me. I suggested he should come over with his sister. In the meantime, the district nurse came and gave Alan an injection, to dry up the saliva secretions. He was more comfortable, and seemed to pick up. I think Michael and Caroline arrived separately. I don't know what time they came. I can't remember exactly. Caroline had brought James with her. They all stayed until the evening.

While we were all with him, Alan tried to say something to us. We went through the letters of the alphabet with him, and he winked when we reached the right letter. Eventually, we managed to work out what he wanted to say which was: 'I can't even die to order.' We laughed. Knowing his sense of humour, we thought he found the scene of us all sitting around his bedside, waiting for him to die, amusing. That was my initial interpretation. But he wasn't laughing. I realised, after it was too late. I realised, as I looked into his eyes. I could see the tears he didn't want anyone to see. His grandson was holding his hand. Alan didn't want to cry. Perhaps it was just as well we all laughed. But he wasn't being funny. The words were poignant.

Whenever I left the room, his eyes would light up the minute I walked back in. I only know this because his daughter said so, and it is the only memory of him with the disease that I don't mind holding on to. Only a few days before, when he was trying to tell me how much he loved me, he said 'I want you to be the last person I see, when I reach the end of my mortal life. You have to know that.' Our last few months together had been so hard, and in so many ways. The disease hadn't let either of us be ourselves. We had both found it difficult. I think that is why he said this to me. He wanted me to be left in no doubt how much I meant to him, right up to the end of his life. I could see it in his eyes. Our love for each other had withstood all the tests life had thrown at us.

But for that moment, he had around him all the people he loved most. He wasn't allowed to die while he had them in his sight.

He was awake before his daughter left, but fell asleep before his son went home. As he seemed to have picked up with the injection, it didn't seem unreasonable to assume that he would still be with us the next day, or even another week. I still thought it was possible he could be with us for some while yet.

The district nurses came back to check on him, but it was too early to give him another injection. They had been trying to arrange a Marie Curie nurse to spend the night with us, so I would be able to get some sleep. But in the end, it didn't happen.

When we were alone, on the evening before he died, I stood at the bottom of his bed thinking, 'If only I could have my Alan back.' The person lying there was so desperate to leave his mortal life behind – to be rid of the disease.

'You do know I love you?' I asked him. I needed to ask him. I had wanted to be an angel for him. I had tried so hard. I had even tried to make miracles happen; anything, but lose him.

Now that it was time to let go, I needed to know he understood the times when I had been anything but an angel. He answered by saying just two words, but two words that let me know he understood: 'you must.'

Knowing how much he wanted to die, but still not wanting him

210

to leave me, I said, 'You will always be in my heart.' He looked at my heart as though he was determined that he would be.

I lay on the bed, in the small space beside him. My right arm was over him. 'I'm sorry it had to end this way,' he said. I heard every single word. This was our fate. I wished it had not been so. We did have a wonderful life together. We had made the best of what life together had given us, but it was not without disappointment along the way. The sorrow was for lost hopes and dreams, as well as for the way our life together had had to end.

'Me too. It has been so cruel.'

'Yes it has.' The end of his life had been so cruel in so many ways.

I connected up Alan's feeding tube to the overnight feed. The district nurses came back to give Alan another injection, last thing. This would hopefully keep him comfortable until the morning.

Knowing he was comfortable, I asked him, 'Is it OK if I go to bed? I am so tired.' 'Yes. You go to bed.'

'You promise you won't die in the night.'

'I won't.' He knew I was tired, and was saying what he thought was best for me. He always did. He was still trying to care for me!

I was tired, but I still wanted to be with him at the very end. I wanted to be there holding him when he died, feeling his warmth for the last time. And if I had been with him, I could have made sure that he didn't suffer, in his last moments. I am fairly sure he died peacefully, in his sleep, but not absolutely sure. I was in the house with him. We were together, but I wasn't there with him, beside him. So I will never be sure.

He asked me not to draw the curtains. He had done the same the night before. I went to bed. Did I kiss him goodnight? I must have. I always did. But I was so tired, I can't remember whether I did or not, and I expected to see him in the morning. Did I kiss him? I have asked myself this question over and over.

One thing I think I can be fairly sure of is what his prayer would have been before he went to sleep. After all, he had told me only recently, that he had prayed every night, before he went to sleep, ever since he was a child. There were so many things I still had to learn about him. He couldn't die now, not yet. But he needed to die. The disease had won. So he would have prayed that night. He would have given thanks for his life. He would have prayed for all those he loved to be looked after, and I am sure he would have finished his prayer with, 'God Bless …' going through each of our names, right through to each of his grandchildren.

25 April 2006

I slept like a log. When I woke up the house was quiet. The sun was shining brightly through the curtains. I got up, pulled the curtains back, and stood for a moment, looking out of the window, and down at the garden. The house felt different, as though something monumental had changed in my life. I went downstairs. I couldn't look at Alan straightaway. I was waiting, hoping he would say 'Ello,' as I walked into the room. But there was only silence.

I looked at him. He was lying there with his eyes closed. He looked so peaceful. I felt relief that his suffering was over.

But part of me was left unsure, uncertain that he had died peacefully. I had been terribly torn when I went to bed, but I was so shattered. I knew there was a chance he would die in the night, but I wanted to be with him when he died, and if someone had stayed with us they could have woken me up. It wasn't that I needed to say good-bye; I simply needed to share his last moment, and be sure that he was allowed to die peacefully, especially as the last part of his life had been anything but kind. And I had missed my chance to tell him how happy he had made me. Yes, I had agreed with him when he said, 'We have had a wonderful life.'

'But this bit has been so hard,' I had added. There had been that word 'but'.

Maybe, not being beside each other in his last moment had spared us in some way. Perhaps it would have been too painful for us. After all, it was the disease we wanted to be rid of – not each other. Perhaps fate was making an effort to be kind, by ensuring we were both asleep: blissfully unaware. I hope he went to sleep when I left him, and simply didn't wake up, but I couldn't be sure. He looked as though he had died that way, but I couldn't be sure. I can never be sure. The disease had gone, but other than this, the only comfort was that he had died at home. We were together in the house, but I was not by his side. Did he die peacefully in his sleep? I can never be sure. I touched his arm. He was still warm. He had kept his promise to me. He had died in the morning. And he had had his wish. I had been the last person he saw in his mortal life.

It was not the life I had once dreamed of, nor could I ever have imagined the way it would turn out. The love we shared, the friendships we enjoyed together, the places we went, his children and grandchildren – everything – enriched my life beyond my dreams. All this, because of one weekend in Cornwall, twenty-six years before, when he had been at a lose end. Alan didn't just add a touch of colour to my life. He added the whole spectrum. I would not have missed it for the world.

Epilogue

We Meet Again

There were two pools side by side – a shallow one and a deep one. I walked along the wide step of one of them, the water lapping over my feet. Suddenly, I realised it wasn't the shallow pool. This frightened me and I lost my balance. I struggled to keep myself from falling into the deep water.

Alan saw it all from where he was sitting, beside the other pool. He came over to me. He knew my fear of the water. He stood behind me. I leaned back into his strong arms and he let me gently down onto the step. I don't know what made me lean back. While I lay there, he held my head with one hand, and stroked my forehead with the other. The water lapped over me. As I lay there, looking up into his face, he was smiling down at me. He looked handsome, as always, but much younger, just as he had looked when we first met. His eyes were twinkling and kind. With him there, I was safe; no thought of drowning entered my head. With him there, I had nothing to fear.

And as I looked into his face, he leaned down towards me. I started to reach up to him, but as I did so he gently pulled me up towards him. We kissed one another gently on the lips, then gently again. As I went to kiss him again, I woke up. It was another dream.

Only Alan knew me well enough to know what these symbols would mean to me. By using them I would know what he was trying to tell me in my dream.

His love will always be with me. I have our memories. In trying to look to the future, I imagine him beside me, saying: 'You can do it', and who knows, maybe he is here in some way, here to share the future with me. When I think of this dream, I can still feel his warmth.

Alan John Wood
1934 to 2006

My rock, my strength, my greatest treasure. I would not have missed this life with you for the world. Until we meet again, Darling Angel, your love will always be in my heart.

Glossary and Information

First Symptoms and Diagnosis

Page 2 - **Atrial flutter** is a type of irregular heartbeat in which the atria (upper chambers of the heart) beat so rapidly that the conducting mechanism, between the atria and the ventricles (lower chambers of the heart), is unable to respond to every beat. As a result, the ventricles beat only once to every two, three or four beats of the atria. Atrial fibrillation is a type of irregular heartbeat in which the atria beat very rapidly, and not all these beats pass through the conducting mechanism between the atria and the ventricles causing the ventricles to beat irregularly.

Page 4 - **MND** is the name given to a small group of related diseases affecting the motor neurones (nerve cells) in the brain and spinal cord. As the motor neurones gradually die, the muscles stop working. This leads to weakness and wasting of the muscles. The cause is, as yet, unknown.

Page 10 - **EMG** is the abbreviation for electromyogram, a recording of the electrical activity in muscles. Small disc electrodes are attached to the skin surface over the muscles or alternatively small needle electrodes are inserted into the muscles to detect electrical impulses.

Page 13 - **Cervical spondylosis** or cervical osteoarthritis is a degenerative disorder that affects the joints between the cervical vertebrae, the bones in the neck.

A Time to Share and a Time to Tell

Page 50 - **Amyotrophic Lateral Sclerosis** (ALS) is the most common type of motor neurone disease. In most cases, the first symptom is weakness in the hands and arms, accompanied by wasting of the muscles.

Preparing for Battle

Page 66 - **Riluzole** was the first drug to be licensed for the treatment of MND. Research suggested that this drug might slow the disease.

Page 74 - **Cardioversion** is a technique in which a brief electric shock is administered to the heart. It is also called defibrillation

Page 82 - **Attendance Allowance** is a tax-free allowance, which is not means-tested. It is for people over the age of 65, who are dependent on others for personal care or mobility

Taking a Chance

Page 106 - **The Oxford Centre for Enablement**, Northfield Orthopaedic Centre NHS Trust, Oxford.

The Trip to China

Page 124 - **Convene** is the brand name of bags that can be used by anyone who finds it difficult to urinate in a toilet. The bag is held in place on the leg and invisible under trousers or skirts.

Fighting the Disease

Page 161 - **Tracheostomy** is an operation to make an opening in the trachea (windpipe) and a tube is inserted to maintain an effective airway. Non–invasive positive pressure ventilation (NPPV) is a mechanical form of ventilation, which works by increasing pressure in a person's airways and thus forcing additional air into the lungs. This is usually done via a mask that fits over the nose and mouth, a bit like an oxygen mask, or only over the nose.

Running Out of Ammunition

Page 189 - **Feeding tubes** are placed with the aid of the scope. The scope goes down the throat to assist in guiding the placement of the tube through the wall of the stomach. The feeding tube extends from the interior of the stomach to outside the body through a small incision, only slightly larger than the tube itself, in the abdominal wall. The tube is prevented from coming out of the stomach by one of several methods. One method employs a very small balloon at the end of the tube that is inflated within the stomach after the insertion.

Till All Our Fight be Fought

Page 206 - **Hyoscine patches** (active ingredient: hyoscine hydrobromide) help by decreasing saliva secretions in the throat. Saliva secretions can be uncomfortable and difficult to clear if swallowing becomes a problem, and in such circumstances patches are easier to administer than tablets.

The Motor Neurone Disease (MND) Association is the only national organisation in England, Wales and Northern Ireland dedicated to the support of people with MND and those who care for them. It works to help people with MND secure the care and support they need; educates and supports health and social care professionals in order to improve the care provided for people living with MND; while promoting research into causes, treatments and a cure.

For more information about MND and the MND Association go to www.mndassociation.org.

MND Connect offers people affected by MND access to a quick route to advice and practical and emotional support. It also provides direction to other services and agencies.

Contact MND Connect on 08457 626262

or

email mndconnect@mndassociation.org.

Seven Arches Publishing will be making a donation to the MND Association from the sale of every book.

Seven Arches Publishing Principles

We are a small publisher that mainly publishes novels for children. Our books for adults are in the memoir genre and general fiction based on life experiences. We have ethical standards that mean we hope our books make a difference.

We are striving to make our business a good place for people to work and to offer employment to those, who through disabilities or other reasons, have found it difficult to get work elsewhere.

Our books are generally printed in this country so that delivery is nearby and the paper used is from managed forests.

Contact Us

You are welcome to contact Seven Arches Publishing by:

Phone: 0161 612 0866

Or

Email: admin@sevenarchespublishing.co.uk

Another Great Read From
Seven Arches Publishing

My Teacher Says You're A Witch
By Jane Schaffer

An inspection is a very public judgement on a school and the impact on head-teachers and staff is well documented but the experience of the inspector is rarely explored. Jane Schaffer does that in this tale of the journey from the teacher's desk at the front of the class-room to the inspector's chair at the back.

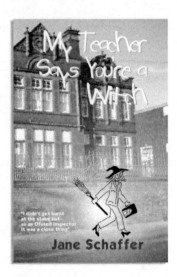

A fictional and often humorous account of life as a schools inspector that captures the very essence of primary education. A must for all teachers, parents and governors.

"I enjoyed it…A sensitive and humane account of school inspection which should be read by all nervous schools and tyro inspectors alike."
Chris Woodhead former Chief Inspector of Schools

"I didn't think I could possibly like a book about Ofsted, but I am enjoying it immensely!"
Christine Anderson, Teacher at Stanley Grove
Primary School, Manchester

Buy this book from our website and pay no postage and packing
www.sevenarchespublishing.co.uk